616.123
NAE

APR 2013

A Woman's Heart Attack:

What Your Doctor May Not Tell You

What Every Women Needs to Know to Prevent,
Recover, and Heal from a Heart Attack

D o r i A . N a e r b o Ph.D.

DISCARD

Lincoln Park Library
7300 Ridgeview Avenue
Pittsburgh, PA 15235

A Woman's Heart Attack: What Your Doctor May Not Tell You. Copyright © 2012 by Dori A. Naerbo, Ph.D. All rights reserved. Printed in the United States of America. No part of this book may be used or reproduced in any manner whatsoever without written permission except in the case of brief quotations embodied in critical articles or reviews.

Author: Dori A. Naerbo, Ph.D

Edited by: Beth Hewett, Ph.D.

ISBN-10: 1477604103

ISBN-13: 978-1477604106

A Note To Readers

This book is for informational purposes only. Readers are advised to consult a physician. The information, ideas and suggestions contained in this book are not intended to serve as a substitute for professional medical advice. Any use of the information or suggestion in this book is at the reader's discretion. The author and publisher specifically disclaim any and all liability arising directly or indirectly for the use or application of any information contained in this book. A health care professional should always be consulted regarding your specific condition or situation.

This book is based on true events, therefore, the author has taken the liberty to change or omit the names in order to protect the privacy of others.

Lincoln Park Library

Dedication

This dedication is to my loving mother who was taken from us much too early. She always supported and believed in me, no matter what it was, she was always my greatest cheerleader.

To my beautiful children Ann, Eric and Kirsten. You are the best and most thoughtful children. You are all truly heaven sent, angels from above. I am so proud of the people you are now and who you will become in the future.

To my husband Kurt, my best friend, my partner, and the love of my life. He has stood by me; he is my rock, my biggest supporter and advocate to help me get this important message out.

To all my fellow sisters, caregivers, and those who have had heart attacks, heart disease, and stem cell therapy, who shared their lives and inspired me to write.

And finally, to the Napoleon Hill Foundation. This was the spark and encouragement I needed to finish one of my life's works.

Contents

Praise For:
A Woman's Heart Attack: What Your Doctor May Not Tell You

"Dr. Naerbo presents a convincing argument acting as an ambassador for the improvement of women's health. I found *A Woman's Heart Attack: What Your Doctor May Not Tell You* to be an illuminating read that will surely inspire many heart patients to become their own best advocate in creating awareness for the number one killer of women, heart disease."

— Amit N. Patel, M.D., B.S., M.S. Associate Professor of Cardiothoracic Surgery at University of Utah

"While folk wisdom has long held that the eyes are the window to one's soul, Dr. Dori Naerbo, masterfully wields words to shine a light on her own. She generously and un-flinchingly shares her truth, and reminds us that with intuition, conviction, determination and faith we have the power to save our own lives. *A Woman's Heart Attack: What Your Doctor May Not Tell You* is a must read for all women who want real help healing hearts, minds and yes, their souls."

—Sher Lipson, MSW, ACSW

"*A Woman's Heart Attack: What Your Doctor May Not Tell You* is about the experience of being a woman. Only great women are able to put a huge mirror in front of us and show us that the way things are is not an inevitable destiny. Dori had the courage to question all that was taken for granted for too long and has been internalized to such deep levels. Dr Dori Naerbo stands near her mirror and reflects on us, with this book, every moment, feeling and action that the experience of being a woman taking her destiny into her own hands may become. Dori is just that great of a woman."

— Nira Kaplansky, Ph. D.
CEO of Waterbirds

"I first became familiar with Dori and her scientific work at the end of our two parallel journeys. I am astonished by the description of Dori's life since she discovered that she was ill and managed to get better on her own aided solely by what God gave her.

As part of this incredible journey, with its difficult parts where things sometimes got bogged down, Dori discovered the connection between body, mind and spirit, and used it to heal herself. She then decided that whatever it takes, she would do her outmost to ensure that more people can benefit from her discoveries and from the methods she developed to check, integrate and optimize one's bodily and mental functions.

A Woman's Heart Attack: What Your Doctor May Not Tell You, provides invaluable insights to optimize your healing potential."

— Yael Porat, Ph.D.
Scientist, Inventor and CEO of BiogenCell

Foreword

Dear Readers,

The first time I met Dr. Dori at our annual Napoleon Hill Foundation Leader Certification Program in Ireland 2011 she appeared the picture of health. Her skin glowed, her hair was thick, dark, and shiny, and her professional style and figure complemented her total look. She appeared stable, secure, and in charge of herself from the inside out. As the days passed during our training, Dori shared a much different story, however. Recently she had suffered three life-threatening heart attacks and was lucky to be alive. Yet, here she was enrolled in this intensive course looking young and vibrant. I wondered how she survived. Next, I wondered how she would follow her stated purpose and disclose her plan of action that totally healed her physically.

An essential part of healing is having the right mental attitude toward becoming whole and healthy. In Dr. Dori A. Naerbo's book *A Woman's Heart Attack: What Your Doctor May Not Tell You*, emphasis is placed upon empowering yourself with accurate medical information while simultaneously conditioning your mind for wholeness and healing. Body, mind, and spirit are the component parts of each individual. Healing is an integral process that needs to incorporate each of these segments. Illness first begins to develop in our ethereal body. Knowing what triggers physical illness is a starting point for anyone desiring to correct the problem when and where it first originates. Life threatening illness as extreme as a heart attack does not just happen without cause. Although the warning signs may be subtle, there are indicators that lead to the event.

Dr. Dori presents her subjective view of what happened to her not once, twice, but three times as she experienced three cardiac infarctions. She counts herself lucky to be alive to detail her personal experience, but more importantly to guide us along the path towards our own care and healing. Life today leaves little to chance. As we become imbalanced in our self-care due to demands made upon us over time, we realize that not only are we compromising our health, but we are neglecting the other avenues that create a well-balanced lifestyle. Knowing what to do and doing it is unfortunately not the same thing. If asked, each of us can recognize what is good for our well-being, and not so good. Oftentimes the answers are evident, but the daily application of healthy choices are not practiced in our day to day living.

Choosing a philosophy or pattern to follow that positions you on the road to improved living may be a place to start. Dr. Dori embraces Napoleon Hill's Philosophy of Success as outlined in the 17 Success Principles that began to take shape with Dr. Hill's premier book *Law of Success* in 1928, advanced in understanding in his classic Think *and Grow Rich* in 1937, and were finalized in Hill's comprehensive course PMA *Science of Success* in the 60s. Over these several decades of case study analysis, Dr. Hill acquired the data to identify 17 Principles or characteristics of successful persons. These characteristics are commonly understood, and when applied actively in a person's life give an individual access to improved conditions for maintaining a positive mental attitude (PMA), a healthy lifestyle, and sound spiritual anchoring for today's world. Mental, physical, emotional, social, spiritual, and financial are all parts of life's riches and need to be addressed as a person seeks balance and well-being in everyday life.

Dr. Dori decides to examine what led up to her sequence of heart attacks, and how she became determined to turn her health around before it became too late to stop the downward spiral. First, she had to understand what happened to her medically and why, and in the same investigative manner, she had to uncover what aspects of her mental and spiritual behavior contributed to her health crisis. She does not look outside herself to place external blame, but rather questions her lifestyle, heredity, state of mind, and actions that led up to her health episodes. Each of us forms our outcome through our day by day practices. This may be done consciously or unconsciously. They key is to uncover what we may be doing unconsciously that may be eroding our conscious actions and preferred outcomes.

Dr. Dori's gift to us is that she reflects on the steps that led to her health crises in order that we might pinpoint some of these same warning signs in our own life. Dr. Dori's gift is one of hindsight that we can incorporate now as foresight in our own lives. If we know what the outcome can become due to similar choices that we recognize from Dori's story, we can prepare ourselves for a better tomorrow by making beneficial choices in time prior to dealing with a physical setback. How often have you stated: "I wish I knew that in advance." Well, now you do, so there is even a better reason to get yourself on the right track before you become derailed by a health crisis that you never even anticipated.

It is with great admiration and appreciation that I acknowledge Dr. Dori's effort in sharing her personal story with each of us. It is through this type of selfless giving that a person such as Dori contributes to making the world a better place in which to live.

In appreciation for your gift, Dori, I acknowledge and commend your heartfelt willingness to freely share your personal story for the benefit of everyone who reads it.

Blessings,

Judy Williamson

Judith Williamson
Director, Napoleon Hill World Learning Center
Purdue University Calumet
September 2012

Preface

At my last cardiovascular visit, my doctor said,
"You've completely healed yourself! I can see no
evidence that you have had a heart attack!"

This book is based on my years of research, observation, and how I completely healed myself; it will challenge everything you think you know about heart attacks in women. Heart disease is the number one killer of women worldwide, find out what makes a woman vulnerable.

After three consecutive heart attacks and with a fourth looming like a dark cloud, I had to take action and figure out why I was sick. I had to stop the next heart attack. Numb, depressed, paralyzed with fear, and frustrated with conventional medicine, I started my quest, determined to solve the problem that no one seemed to be able to answer for me. *A Woman's Heart Attack: What Your Doctor May Not Tell You* is a story of my healing journey and the specific steps I took to heal myself.

Early into my research about my heart disease, I began to realize that I needed to use my body, mind, and spirit as one for healing to occur. For this reason, *A Woman's Heart Attack: What Your Doctor May Not Tell You* is divided into three parts, which address the body, mind, and spirit. I teach you step by step what I did to achieve healing and good health after surviving my heart attacks. The journey to health is truly remarkable. You will learn some of the patterns that happen before a heart attack, the relationship between hormones and heart attacks, gender differences between women's and men's heart disease, how to prevent the next attack, and how to heal yourself.

I started writing this book in 2005 as part of my own healing therapy, but later it grew into something much more and I realized that what I learned could help all women. This book became a guide to self healing and enlightenment. After my doctor told me the good news of my fully healed heart, I knew it was time to complete the book and share what I did to bring about new heart health to all women. My hope is that *A Woman's Heart Attack: What Your Doctor May Not Tell You* will help you in your quest for a healthy heart and the improved quality of life that comes along with it.

Prelude

❤ Women's heart attacks are different from men's—both in why they occur and how they are experienced.

❤ We have the ability to transform our health both negatively and positively. I hope you will want to develop good health for yourself.

❤ Having a heart attack is devastating and it can feel like the end of the world, but there is hope. A heart attack has an impact on the body, mind, and spirit—each of which needs our assistance to heal.

❤ We live in an age where we can create a health care team that works for each of us on an individual level. Build your medical care team with such health care professionals as an internist, cardiologist, allopath, nutritionist/dietician, exercise specialist, psychologist, coach, and spiritual advisor.

Four Life Challenges

When I was forty-seven years old, I had three consecutive heart attacks—during the months of July, August, and September of 2005. Why were these attacks occurring? How did I come to be in such precarious health? I felt well enough and was unaware of any heart problems before these attacks. Just as much to the point, how did I come not only to survive these attacks but also to become—in my doctor's words—"completely healed" and certainly well enough to write a book about my experiences?

My health was challenged, I think, by several life changes that occurred over a five-year period. My first change involved a move from California across the Atlantic Ocean to Europe. Kurt, my Norwegian husband of fifteen years at the time, and I moved our family from California to Norway. This was a major life event, not only for me but our teenaged children. Our three children were Ann, fourteen; Eric, twelve; and Kirsten, seven. Uprooting them was difficult, but we persuaded Ann in particular, who was just entering high school, that she would someday think this move to be one of the best opportunities of her life.

It was bittersweet leaving our home in Fallbrook, where we had lived for fifteen years. Until that move, Kurt and I had spent our entire married life in that house. We built it ourselves, and it was an expression of us. I had all my babies, all the family get-togethers—every event in my married life—occurred within those walls. That home represented my accumulated hopes and perceived future.

The three-story house, surrounded by remarkably shady palm trees, boasted a healthy lawn, spacious rooms, and all the sunshine we needed to raise our children. It was gut-wrenching and bittersweet as we drove away, yet, I remained positive about our new journey in life. The girls and I sobbed as we said our farewells and waved goodbye to our familiar home. It was a sad day, and my heart was heavy. Even though, I know it's just a house, a shell, a casing, nothing more, I still have trouble looking at pictures without missing it, but time has a way of softening painful memories. As we left, I reminded the girls that being a family is more important than where the family lives. We were on our way to join Kurt and Eric, who were already in Norway waiting for us. My friends thought I was crazy for leaving, but Kurt was homesick and I had promised that I would consider living in Norway. I decided that it didn't matter where we lived; I could make any house our home as long as we were together.

There is a silver lining in everything if we can just open our eyes, take the blinders of our past dreams off for a few seconds, and allow our perspectives to change. That's one of this book's messages. I chose to see my glass as have full, not have empty. Yes, it was challenging to leave and start over, but *life is an adventure*. In 1998, we remade our life in Norway. I was a high-powered American executive living in a foreign country, and I could not speak Norwegian except for rudimentary phrases. I knew just enough for basic interactions. Without friends or a phone, I struggled to get my family settled. Home base was a rental house, where it was colder than I ever dreamed possible, far from sunny California. I felt frozen. Looking at our situation, I thought: "Oh my God, what have I done?"

Rather than wallowing in confusion, I chose to make positive changes to improve my situation. I needed to learn Norwegian. Practicing with tapes and a class did not work for me, so I learned the language by immersing myself into the culture and landed a dream job working for a premier management and IT consulting firm. My work involved IT security, life science, and global knowledge management responsibilities for eight countries. It challenged and electrified me. Life in Norway was like a fairytale, Kurt thrived, the children adapted and made new friends, and I felt valued once again. We actually had time to be a real family.

However, the fairytale came to an end a few years later and within three months, three more life changes happened so quickly that I did not recognize their complex challenges until well after they occurred.

In the first event, my job happiness simply didn't last; the terrorist events of September 11, 2001 not only stunned our family, but also impacted the service line of my company. Consequently, my division was disbanded in 2002. I accepted the offered severance package, feeling confident and certain that I would find another job easily. I did not. In Norway, a worker over age forty-five is considered somewhat old.

The final two major life events were the worst that I experienced. Shortly after I lost my job and just before Christmas that year, my brother Donny died. Four days later, my mother died. I had to return to the United States to prepare a double funeral. The deaths of my mother and brother in such a short time devastated me. The double portion of grief, compounded by my family's grief, disarmed me and eroded any strength that had been shielding me. These deaths were the second and third major life events. They were also the most devastating.

Over the course of two more years, I searched for the perfect job. I wondered what my life's purpose might be. Since my children were nearly grown, I wanted my job to be my calling in life and to leave my mark, my legacy in the world. But what was that vocation and legacy? What was my specific purpose in life? I love medicine and technology, but a desire to help people and make a difference for them also churned inside me. The twin loves pulled me in competing directions, so I struggled to clarify what I genuinely wanted to do. My aimless job search almost certainly contributed to stress in my life.

Heart Problems

In May 2005, I came down with whooping cough even though I was vaccinated as a child. The doctors told me that my youngest daughter Kirsten had infected me. She tested positive despite having received the vaccination as a toddler. When I asked about antibiotics, my doctor said no. She said I would be coughing for about three months. I thought: *You have got to be kidding! I cannot cough like this for three months. I can see why whooping cough kills babies and small children.* Coughing jags felt like strangulation. They left me exhausted and required at least twenty minutes of rest to catch my breath.

A few months later, my heart health suffered the effects of all those stressors. I experienced two definitive heart attacks, one in July and another in August. In September, I had a heart event that was one test number away from being defined as a third heart attack. My doctor said something was happening to my heart, but the attack wasn't strong enough for me to be hospitalized; yet, to me, the event clearly *was* a third attack. The cardiologists were stumped. They gave me drugs and sent me on my way with utterly no instructions about preventing future heart attacks and no explanation for why I had the heart attacks in the first place.

I was familiar with heart problems from my father. His heart was so sick that eventually he needed a heart transplant. But I didn't have the heart disease that he had. It was a mystery. I was a forty-seven-year old, healthy and life-loving woman with a very sick heart. I needed to understand why, but the doctors could not tell me. They gave me no reasons and no reassurance. Not knowing was unacceptable to me and it led me to my quest, which was to find my own answers.

A Quest for Answers

I decided to document my observation, just as if I were in a hospital setting and medical personnel were charting. I figured that they would create a daily charting of my bodily functions, nutritional intake, symptoms, and medications, which is exactly what I started to make. In Chapter Five, I explain how in detail. This daily activity enabled me to find the pattern that would lead to my own healing. I believe that everything has a pattern; we just need to find it. To me, medications address the symptoms rather than a cure. Please note that I'm not saying you shouldn't take the medications ordered by a health care provider: I'm saying you should understand why they are needed. More importantly, we need to find out the cause of the problem instead of just treating its symptoms.

Our bodies, minds, and spirits are connected in profound ways that can cause us to become ill or help us to get well. I decided to take a positive thinking approach to my heart health, and in doing so, I took charge of my life. The body is an amazing piece of machinery, but our minds — conscious and subconscious — and spiritual lives are enmeshed with it to create whole and unique persons. I knew that even though my father had a heart attack, a quintuple bypass, and a heart transplant back in the early 1980s, my fate didn't have to be the same as his. Since I refused to accept this, I took my mind and spirit on a quest to figure out what was wrong with my body, which led to my complete recovery. In fact, my cardiologist said: "You have completely healed yourself. I can't see any evidence that you ever had a heart attack!"

This book recognizes that all of us are unique. What works for some may not work for others. Listen to your body. You know how from other experiences in your life. For example, a doctor once prescribed antibiotics for one of my children. Within a few minutes, my child started projectile vomiting. My mind immediately jumped to an allergy, but my doctor insisted I force the medication down her throat. She ended up in the hospital two days later with a severe loss of blood platelets, meaning that a vital organ could hemorrhage. I told myself after that horror that I would listen to the body's cues from then on.

After my second heart attack, I was reminded of this near accident with my daughter. I was angry because I was the perfect, complaint patient; I followed all directions. I took all my medications like a good patient only to have a second heart attack worse than the first. The doctors gave me the maximum dose of Lipitor, and I didn't even have a cholesterol problem. My cholesterol levels were excellent. I knew when I took that medicine it was unsuitable for my body. I could barely walk, breathe, or do anything else. But the doctors prescribed it to me, and I thought they knew better. Soon, life literally felt like it was not worth living. I told my husband that if I had to take that pill, I would rather be dead. He was shocked to hear me say those words. My family was worried and constantly watching over me. I looked grave and had large black circles under my eyes. My life force felt like it was slipping away. All I knew was that this cholesterol-reducing drug was making me sick. I was at a crossroad and needed to make a decision whether or not to take the drug.

At this point, I was frustrated with allopathic (traditional) medicine and started looking at nontraditional medicine and nutritional supplementation. While the Internet became my good friend in my search given that books and peer reviewed journals written in English are not easily found in Norway, the Internet also can be a foreboding place when you're sick. Read with a skeptical eye. This is where family, friends, and health advocates are helpful, even necessary. My cardiologists from the hospital dismissed my ideas because nutritional supplements are not scientifically proven drugs. My experience has been that this attitude is as common in the United States as it is in Norway. Eventually, I turned to Dr. Steven Sinatra because he is a cardiologist who understands nutritional needs.

In retrospect, one of the most significant things I did to bring about healing was to apply Napoleon Hill's *Science of Success*, developed in the 1960's. There are seventeen principles, which he realized were beneficial to people in various walks of life after he interviewed successful individuals like John D. Rockefeller, Thomas Edison, and Alexander Graham Bell. These principles struck me as so helpful that I wove them throughout this book. They provide the focus of Chapter Eight's foundations for healing. They've simply become a part of the way I think and act. In other words, I apply these principles to guide my mind and spirit, and in turn, they have influenced my body's health. You can use them to achieve your heart's desire and good health. While I was in graduate school for my Ph.D. in Clinical Psychology I had a successful practice as a clinical hypnotherapist. I would tell my clients that they should *"get to the heart of the matter"* and *"Whatever your mind can conceive and believe it can achieve."* Hill's words have helped me achieve my heart's desires, which are good heart health and a new direction in my life.

My new direction in life is continued work in medical science as an educator, researcher, and patient care advocate in the field of autologous stem cell (ASC) transplantation. I advocate and assist heart patients in determining whether the use of their own stem cells might be an appropriate treatment for their heart diseases. This work, which came about only because of my own heart attacks, has opened new worlds to me and has allowed me to be a positive mentor in other heart patients' lives.

My heart attack experiences and my resulting action for health motivated me to write this book — to share my knowledge and to help other women. Four years later, I'm fully healed.

Since I now work in the field of stem cell research, I speak to thousands of cardiac patients who have asked me to share my experiences. To that end, I'm dedicating this book to my patients, family, and close friends for their emotional support throughout some rough years. And I dedicate it to all the women who will have heart attacks and will want to become well again.

Disclaimers

In a book like this, it is necessary to state what the book doesn't do as well as what it does do. I provide a few disclaimers below.

Health Care Systems

It's important to note that the health care systems of the United States and Norway are hugely different in terms of how they are conceived and carried out. While many American citizens currently pay for health insurance to access health care, Norwegians participate in a centralized health care system. It's called the National Insurance Scheme, and the word "scheme" simply means "plan." The health care system is universally available to all citizens, is tax-funded, and is a single-payer health system, which means that every patient receives the same standard of care. Readers may be curious as to how Norway and the U. S. compare in terms of quality of care. I can only say that I had excellent heart-health care experiences in Norway. I think that some of the issues I encountered in the hospital and with individual health care personnel could have happened in any hospital with any doctors or nurses regardless of the developed country.

This book is not intended to indict or promote one health care system over the other, nor is it a political statement about health care insurance, payment plans, and/or generalized or specific problems. That said, I believe my story can serve as a cautionary tale in many developed countries today. It always behooves us as patients—and as women—to find out as much as possible about an illness and to be an informed partner with our health care providers. We need to be our own advocates and, when possible, we need to recruit family and friends to advocate for us. And, of course, in the unusual situation of not being a completely fluent language speaker in the country where the care is provided, it's essential to speak with health care professionals who are fluent in one's home language in order to understand all the issues connected to the condition and to become well.

About Medical Information

This information is intended as an educational resource only and should not be used for diagnosing or treating a health problem. It's not a substitute for expert professional care. The information and reference materials contained here are intended solely for the general information of the reader. It's not to be used for treatment purposes, but rather for discussion with your own physician. The information contained herein is neither intended to dictate what constitutes reasonable, appropriate, or best care for any given health issue, nor is it intended to be used as a substitute for the independent judgment of a physician for any given health issue. Please consult your health care provider if you have persistent health problems and/or questions.

About Medical Advice

This information is not to be considered medical advice and is not intended to replace consultation with a qualified medical professional. The primary responsibility of your disease management plan is with your treating physicians, and you should only follow your treating physician's advice. Please do not change or modify your disease management plan on your own without consulting your treating physicians.

About Endorsement

Reference to any products, services, hypertext link to the third parties, or other information by trade name, trademark, and supplier or otherwise does not constitute or imply its endorsement, sponsorship, or recommendation. Such references provide examples that have worked for the author.

About Links

Links are provided only as an informational resource. These links are provided simply as a service, and it should not be implied that the author recommends, endorses, or approves of any of the content, nor is the author responsible for their availability, accuracy, or content.

PART ONE

THE PHYSICAL JOURNEY

ONE
CHAPTER

My First Heart Attack

A heart attack is a traumatic experience, and my first heart attack caught me off guard. This chapter tells the story of my first heart attack to set the story for the rest of this book. But more important, my experiences—while unique to me—are used here to teach some of the basics of heart attack symptoms; hospital treatment protocol; and the body, mind, and spirit's reactions to a heart attack. One focus of this chapter, as in this entire book, is to point out ways that women are different from men in their heart attacks and reactions to them.

The First Attack

July 1, 2005—it was 8:00 AM on a lovely, sunny day. The ocean view outside our house was peaceful, as boats plied their way on the water. Kurt and I were getting ready to eat breakfast. Suddenly, I felt a sharp, stabbing pain on the left side of my chest, making it difficult to breathe. (I had felt similar pain as a younger adult. It was something called precordial catch syndrome (PCS). Many mistake this pain for a heart attack.) Then, I felt an uncomfortable lump the size of a golf ball in the center of my sternum, similar to indigestion, which is not a symptom of PCS.

I said to Kurt, "I never get indigestion."

He replied, "You just need to eat something."

Then, I started to experience a strange sensation of not feeling well; it was an odd feeling to explain to Kurt. It seemed like a feeling of impending doom, as if a wave had come over me. I was fine one minute, and then I wasn't. I went upstairs to change from nightclothes, and when I came back down, I was completely exhausted and breathless. I remember thinking, *why am I so out of breath?* As I came into the kitchen, my arms felt heavy. The lump in my chest now had transformed into a burning sensation that extended outward from the center and toward both shoulders. This sensation felt like becoming extremely upset and holding everything in or like jogging up a hill and getting lactic acid buildup in the chest.

Kurt grew anxious and said, "Maybe you should call the doctor." I could see by the look on his face that he was particularly concerned, and something was dreadfully wrong.

When I called, the receptionist said, "Oh, I'm sorry, but your doctor is not in today."

When I told her that I needed to get in to the office that day, she replied, "How about 2:00?"

I was speaking in Norwegian, not my native language, of course. At her reply, I thought: *Good God. Doesn't she hear what I'm saying? Doesn't she understand the seriousness of my situation?* So, in frustration, I blurted out in English: "I could be dead if I have to wait until 2:00! I'm having chest pain!"

That got her attention. "Okay. Come at once."

Not long after I got to the office, the attending physician hooked me to an electrocardiogram (EKG), which monitors the electrical activity in the heart. He immediately said, "You are going to the hospital."

I said: "No. I'm starting to feel better now."

"Well, it's your choice, but I highly recommend it," replied the doctor. At this point, I almost had him convinced that I didn't need to go. How stupid was that? But, it's not unusual for normally healthy people to downplay their symptoms when they suspect that those symptoms might be serious.

Once I agreed to go to the hospital, and an ambulance was dispatched, the doctor tried to insert a peripheral venous catheter (PVC)[1] in my hand to provide quick access to a vein. Unfortunately, inserting the PVC wasn't his best skill, and my veins are relatively small. First, he started with my left hand. He failed and left a painful, colorful lump that were shades of black and blue on that hand. Next, he moved to my right forearm. The nurse in the background watched in horror as the doctor botched the next stick.

I cried out, "That's enough!"

---

1 This particular type of IV was a peripheral venous catheter, or a PVC. Sometimes a PVC is called a peripheral venous line, peripheral venous access catheter, or peripheral IV.

He replied: "Oh, but we must. It's protocol for your admittance to the hospital." *You've got to be kidding*, I thought. *I need a PVC to gain admittance to the hospital?* I said: "This is your last chance. If you don't get that needle in, I'm going to the hospital without it." I wanted to punch him.

After being stuck twenty times during one hospital procedure in America, I had developed an aversion to needles, which only makes the procedure more difficult because fear itself can affect veins to constrict by activating the sympathetic nervous system (Johnstone, 1976). Here's what I've learned to make needle sticks easier:

Ask for a pediatric anesthesiologist or someone in anesthesiology to make the stick.

- ❤ Ask to have the site numbed up with an analgesic cream.
- ❤ Ask for a smaller gauge needle.
- ❤ Get hydrated by drinking water, if allowed.

By the time the ambulance got me to the hospital, my symptoms were almost gone, and I had thought I would be going right back home. No such luck. We had to wait for the cardiac enzyme test to measure troponin (TnT) levels. Troponin is a protein that helps muscles contract. When muscle or heart cells are injured, troponin leaks out, and its levels in the blood rise — confirming a heart attack. There are other cardiac-specific tests as well (i.e., CK, CK-MB, myoglobin, hs-CRP, BNP, and NT Pro BNP), as shown in the chart in this chapter's *Lessons Learned*.

I was confident that I didn't have a myocardial infarction (MI), or heart attack and that these precautions were unnecessary. As women, we tend to down play these things. I knew true heart problems from my father's experience. There was no way that I was sick like that! Indeed, later that day, I was lying in a bed in the hospital hallway, because they didn't have an available room. I told myself that my situation couldn't be very serious if the hospital didn't even have a room for me.

During those long hours, I met a wonderful nurse who took exceptional care of me. When she came with a shot for me, I said, "What is this?" She told me it was an injection to thin out my blood called fractionated heparin. She said, "Okay, I need you to lift up your shirt, and I am going to put this needle in your belly." I was thinking that there was no way I would allow the nurse to inject me in my belly area. But she bent down and gave me a strong, stern look that dared me to argue with her. I thoroughly enjoyed her, she was a powerhouse. The needle stick wasn't bad, but the medicine burned as it was injected. After several of these injections, I learned that it did not burn as much if the needle was placed slightly on a slant.

After several hours of waiting, the hospital found a five-patient per room accommodation for me in the geriatric ward; it certainly wasn't a five-star setting! I had four elderly roommates, none of whom spoke English.

Later that afternoon, the nurse and the doctor came into the room to give me my test results. They approached my bed and sat down beside me; with the nurse on my left side and the doctor on my right. They told me that the cardiac enzyme test showed I had suffered a mild heart attack. *What? Whoa! My mind is not hearing this correctly.* "Excuse me?" Suddenly, time seemed to move in slow motion. This news was not what I expected or wanted to hear. I wanted to hear that I was fine and that the episode of not feeling well was simply nothing, but they weren't saying that. I felt overloaded and out of synch with the world. "Okay," Bewildered at what I am hearing, I said. "I'm sorry. Could you repeat that?"

I heard those dreaded words again. "You have suffered a small heart attack," she said. *Oh, my God. I can't believe what I'm hearing.* I tried to push back the tears, but my eyes were like leaky faucets; they wouldn't stop dripping. I could feel my emotions building up and knew that the dam was going to crack open. *I can't believe it! This is a bad dream. This just can't be happening.* I was stunned and in shock.

They told me how lucky I was to have caught it in time and that they usually do not see patients with such a mild heart attack. I explained that, in California, I was an EMT-D, and worked in the ER, so I knew what to say to get the appropriate level of care. Today cardiac enzyme testing is more sensitive than 20 years ago, and a mild heart attack would have been undetected.

Shortly after getting the news, Kurt came into my room with a new DVD player. He immediately saw that I had been sobbing and asked, "What's happened?"

I said, "They just told me that I had a heart attack!" I choked up again and started crying. This news was just too unbelievable. Yet I had to start believing it. The nurse told me that I wasn't allowed to get out of bed even to go to the bathroom. Since I felt fine at that point, the precaution seemed ridiculous. Their seriousness about staying in bed and using a bedpan when the bathroom was less than ten steps away began to poke a hole through my shock and unbelief and I started to understand that I was, indeed, sick.

Later that evening, after Kurt went home, and the lights were dimmed; the night nurse came to my bed and asked if I wanted a sleeping pill. I was thinking, *Hmm, I don't do drugs. Why would I want a sleeping pill?* I refused the medication. Hours later, at 1:00 AM, I was still wide awake. An elderly woman across the room from me suffered from dementia and kept saying in a little voice, "Heeelloo, are you there?" She called out a dozen times. Finally, I decided that I couldn't get any sleep, and I called for the nurse to ask her to take care of that poor woman and to say that, yes, thank you very much, I'll take that sleeping pill now.

An Angiography

The next day was uneventful since it was the weekend. The cardiologists were trying to schedule me for an angiography, which is a procedure that uses imaging technology to see the inside of blood vessels and organs. It's especially useful for visualizing the interior of the arteries, veins, and heart chambers. I was terrified of this procedure, and just the thought of a catheter threaded up my femoral artery—located in the groin—made me shudder.

In retrospect, I was so apprehensive and fearful of the angiography in part because my father had to lay flat for eight hours after he had the procedure. I remember how uncomfortable and painful it was for him. Another reason was that a family friend who needed an angiography died on the table during the procedure. I was acutely aware of the various risks of this test, which carries a 1.8%-2.0% mortality_rate. Even this small risk felt too high to me, and I was worried. I thought: *Why can't I just have a cardiac MRI or a 64-slice cardiac CT, either of which are less invasive? This is really stressing me out.* Nonetheless, the nurses assured me that the doctor had done thousands of them successfully. In this hospital, I wasn't given any kind of informed consent or anything to sign. That seemed unbelievable, and it set my nerves further on edge.

I was extremely stressed about that procedure, which didn't lead to a good frame of mind for undergoing it. The problem was, of course, that I knew too much. Since the time I was seventeen years old, I had learned a great deal about the heart from my father's experiences: from his heart attack to his bypass surgery to his eventual heart transplant. I witnessed his living hell during those years, and I stood by him when—in fear of all those invasive procedures—he had them all. But, I also knew too little about my own situation, so my memories of my father's medical suffering exacerbated my own fears about my heart troubles — which were completely unannounced and unknown until the day before.

In the evening of my second day in the hospital, the night nurse again asked, "Would you like a sleeping pill?"

As before, I replied, "No thank you." I was as reluctant as ever to take medication. Later that night, the roommate right next to me had foul gas problems with only a curtain to separate us. The woman with dementia started chanting for help, annoying everyone; even the nurses trooped in and out to quiet her down. *How am I going to get some sleep like this? Okay, it's 2:00 AM. Yes, please, I'll take a sleeping pill.*

On Monday, everyone was in a frenzy. The charge nurse seemed distracted, which didn't inspire much confidence. Both my gassy neighbor and I were supposed to have the angiography. Suddenly, the head nurse, who seemed disorganized, was flipping all of her chart pages turned to tell us that we could have breakfast. "What?" I questioned. "We're supposed to be scheduled to have a coronary angiography."

"Oh?" she said, lifting her eyebrows questioningly. Then she looked extremely nervous, shuffling papers, while simultaneously dispensing medications. Wary, I checked my medications to be sure she gave me the right ones. Soon, she returned to the room and said, "Okay, one of you is going down for the angiography." Luckily, it wasn't me going first. So, she told me that I could eat breakfast, but now it was 9:15AM and breakfast was no longer being served.

Before lunch, the doctor arrived to tell me that there was a chance that I might have the procedure later that day, which meant I was to eat only a light lunch. Hours later, still hungry, dinner rolled right by me. Finally, the nurse told me that I would not have a procedure that day, so I had missed dinner, too. *Hmm, this is a good diet*, I thought. I had to wait for the evening snack, by which time I felt starved.

Later that night, before I went to bed, a nurse handed me a brochure that explained the details of the angiography. This pamphlet was the first useful information I had received. However, no one took the time to sit down and explain anything to me. In the USA it is normal and customary to inform patients about procedures and sign consent forms, but in Norway, this is not done. My discomfort is based on my previous experience with hospitals in the USA, whereas a Norwegian patient would never think twice about informed consent. Although, on one level, I already knew and understood the information, but that was from my perspective as a daughter and it felt different as the patient. I knew I could deal with procedures when they are done for someone else—no problem. But I found that I wanted a little hand holding when it came to preparing for my own procedure. I felt vulnerable, and yes, I was scared.

On Tuesday morning, July 5, I woke early to wait for my angiography. Today the nurse told me that she wasn't sure whether I was on the list of scheduled patients, so I was allowed to have a very light breakfast. Later that afternoon, my favorite nurse, popped in to tell me that it was time. I started stressing, and I felt the tears welling up in my eyes. She looked straight into my eyes with sincerity and compassion, and said, "You'll be okay. I'll see you back upstairs when it's over." My stress level started to disappear as I found comfort in her words.

It's hard to explain how much I dreaded that procedure. The doctor gave me sedatives to calm my nerves. My body has a tendency to metabolize anesthesia and sedatives rapidly, especially when I'm under stress. Although, I felt the tension drain away quickly, I knew the effects would not be long lasting. I have always been like this; for example, when I had my last child by a cesarean section, I felt everything even under general anesthesia.

That experience was a living nightmare. At the time my doctors said the reason that this happened was due to my heighten sense of awareness. Regardless, I knew the procedure needed to proceed promptly and efficiently in order to avoid pain and keep me calm.

As it happens with so many anxieties in life, the angiography was not nearly as bad as my expectation of it. The worst part for me was the pain of lying flat and still on my back with straight legs for four to six hours after the procedure. Happily, the results were outstanding. My coronary arteries were clear of obstructions, and I didn't need to have any stents, which are tubes inserted into the arteries to restore blood flow. Everything appeared normal. That was the good news. The frustrating news was that we still didn't know why I had the heart attack.

When I returned to my room just as dinner was being served, I felt starved because I didn't have lunch. I couldn't sit up right away, though, and the nurse told me that she could leave the food in the refrigerator and warm it up when I was ready. Four hours later, I asked for my dinner plate and was told by the night nurse that hospital policy does not allow food to be reheated after two hours. I grumbled something about not being given the right information the first time. However, she prepared a couple of slices of bread with some cold cuts, a typical European small meal. Frankly, I was happy just to have anything. Feeling better, I was able to sleep for the first time in days. I noticed the hospital did not have any specific dietary meals, which I found surprising. Everyone eats the same food, typically, high in sodium.

Women and Angiography

Clearly, there are differences between men and woman, and those differences crop up in more ways than communication styles. Heart problems present differently, too. Traditionally, much medical research has been conducted on the male heart, and many doctors have learned in medical school how to think about the male heart first and foremost. Additionally, many people assume that women don't have the kind of heart problems that men do. According to Dr. Ian Graham, Professor of Cardiovascular Medicine at Trinity College, Ireland, "For a long time we thought women were at lower risk than men." However, he continued, "Women may actually have more severe atherosclerosis, even if they have apparently normal findings on an angiogram." In fact, five years after their first heart attack, research indicates that more women than men will have died from heart disease.

Women especially need to educate themselves about such possibilities. Even though my angiography was in the normal range, it wasn't a cause for rejoicing. Recent research has shown that women who had heart attacks and who were found to have apparently "normal" coronary arteries are at a significant risk for acute heart problems the following year. In fact, women are three times more likely to have normal angiograms than men and, of those individuals with normal angiograms; women are three times more likely to be hospitalized for heart problems than men (Laino, 2005). For that reason, having a "normal" angiogram, means that additional tests need to be done; any complacency on the medical professional's role should not be accepted. Additional tests include checking for microvascular dysfunction or disease of the small heart arteries and conducting such tests as:

❤ Intravascular ultrasound, which uses a catheter and a miniature ultrasound probe.

❤ Dobutamine stress echocardiography, which uses medication to show the heart muscle under stress.

❤ Myocardial infusion imaging, which uses a low dose of radioactive medicine to trace the blood through the arteries, veins, and the heart itself.

Discharge from the Hospital

After a week, I was discharged. Despite what seemed like a chaotic entry into the hospital on the day of my heart attack, I had excellent care in the Norwegian hospital. I was both surprised and pleased since medical care was always one of my concerns about living in a foreign country. In fact, socialized medicine was one of my greatest concerns moving from California to Norway. No surprise because in school we were taught that socialism in general was the next step to communism, and socialized medicine is a bad thing, which is completely ignorant. It's upsetting enough to get sick, but getting sick in a foreign country can be particularly daunting. I found it reassuring to know that the medical care in Norway could be as good as in my home country. And, because Norway has a centralized health care system, my part of the hospital bill — including medications — was only one-hundred dollars. Let me put it into perspective for the same type of services I received in Norway; in the USA it would cost well over fifty thousand dollars and this does not include indirect costs, which could exceed hundreds of thousands of dollars.

Upon discharge, my report revealed that I had an acute non-Q wave infarction, which means that my heart attack may have been caused by a nominally occluded (blocked) artery with a potential for a subsequent heart event. My EKG had been normal. The angiography showed normal coronary (heart) arteries. Although the test could not rule out changes in the heart's walls intersecting at the 1.diagonal branch and the 1. marginal branch, there was no stenosis (narrowing of the blood vessels) that needed treatment. Although the arteries appeared to be normal, the doctors decided to give me antithrombotic treatment for a period of time because they could not rule out blood clots. The treatment was prophylactic in that if blood clots were my problem, the medication would protect against another heart attack. In truth, though, they didn't know why my heart was sick.

Using standard heart disease protocols, they prescribed a number of drugs designed to help prevent a future heart attack. These included:

- ♥ Albyl-E (a form of Acetylsalicylic Acid, or aspirin to thin the blood),

- ♥ Plavix (a powerful prescription blood thinner),

- ♥ Zocor (a cholesterol-lowering medication), and

- ♥ Cozaar Comp or Cozaar Plus (a diuretic and blood pressure-lowering medication).[2]

For someone who prided herself on never taking medication, I was overwhelmed with these prescriptions. Being told to take all of these drugs practically screamed *"you're sick!"* to me, and it depressed me. Armed with my new medications, I went home, hoping never to return to the hospital. Once home, it took me two weeks to get back on my feet again. I rested a lot and felt weak and easily fatigued for a while. So, I signed up for membership at the local gym and started training six days a week. I saw some improvement in my strength and overall endurance pretty quickly. I was beginning to feel well again.

---

2 Some of these drugs like Albyl-E and Levaxin have different names and/or ingredients in America, but are common to American heart disease treatments.

Lessons Learned

1. Are you having indigestion/heartburn or a heart attack? Trust your gut feelings and not your head. Over thinking the sensations in your body can do grave damage to your heart. If you feel as if something is not right, consider this to be an early warning sign. Immediately go to your doctor or to an emergency room and get checked. I almost talked myself out of going, but I saved my own life by not rationalizing my symptoms.

2. If you have problems with an IV or PVC, ask:

   a) For a pediatric anesthesiologist or someone in anesthesiology to do the stick.

   b) To have the site numbed up with an analgesic cream.

   c) For a smaller gauge needle.

   d) For water to hydrate your body.

3. Research indicates that women who had a heart attack and who were found to have apparently "normal" coronary arteries are at a significant risk for acute heart problems in the following year. Having a "normal" angiogram after a heart attack does not mean that everything is satisfactory. It means that further tests are needed.

4. At discharge:

   a) Have someone with you to ask questions and understand how to take your medications.

   b) Get all your instructions in writing.

c) Get contact numbers for all medical persons involved in your case.

d) Ask for copies of your records.

5. Find out what tests you have received and what they mean. For example, ask about your cardiac biomarkers. The most common test is for cardiac enzymes to assess troponin (TnT) levels. This is an indication that confirms a heart attack. Other tests include the CK, CK-MB, myoglobin, hs-CRP, and BNP and NT Pro BNP.

Cardiac Test	What It Is	What It Shows	When It Is Given
cTnT (Cardiac Troponin T and Troponin I)	Regulatory proteins that control the calcium-mediated action between the myosin and actin in cardiac muscle.	During a heart attack, tissue dies, and myocardial necrosis cardiac troponins are released.	This test is used within 2-8 hours of the suspected MI and then repeated until the numbers drop to normal.
CK (Creatine Kinase or Creatine Phosphokinase)	An enzyme found in the heart and other tissues.	CK rises in the blood when muscle or heart cells are damaged.	This test is given diagnostically and repeated every 4-6 hours. Three tests are usually given.
CK-MB (Creatine Kinase-MB)	An enzyme found only in the heart.	CK-MB is sensitive to the heart muscle, and it rises when there is damage to the heart even if there are no other signs of heart attack.	This test can be given within 3-4 hours after the onset of chest pain. The concentration peaks in 18-24 hours and then returns to normal within 72 hours.

Myoglobin	A protein in the heart and muscles.	When there is damage to the heart, myoglobin is released into the blood.	This test can be given within 2-3 hours of a heart attack. It peaks within 8-12 hours and usually falls back to normal within one day.
hs-CRP (High-Sensitivity C-Reactive Protein)	A marker for inflammation.	The hs-CRP test can accurately detect lower concentrations of the protein because it's most sensitive.	This test is used to determine cardiovascular risk profile.
BNP and NT Pro BNP (Brain Natriuretic Peptide; proBNP)	A healthy heart normally produces low levels of a precursor protein, called pro-BNP.	BNP and NT-proBNP are produced mainly in the heart's left ventricle. When the heart is overworking and is beyond its capacity, BNP can be detected.	This test is used to rule out heart failure. It's an important analysis that indicates cardio-renal distress.

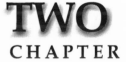

CHAPTER

My Second and Third Heart Attacks

I had no reason to suspect that I would have a second and even a third heart attack, but I was afraid of them anyway. When they occurred, they upset me more than I could have imagined. These two heart events took me deeper into the world of heart health and showed me that I needed to fight an onset of depression and take charge of my health in order to get better. These are actions that I encourage readers to do for themselves.

A Second Attack

Six weeks after I left the hospital, I thought I was doing much better—I had more energy and was becoming comfortable on my medication regimen. Although one month earlier, I complained to my primary doctor about heart palpitations, thoughts of my heart attack were fading, and life was getting back to normal.

Suddenly, at 5:30 PM on August 19, 2005, I felt a flushing throughout my body. I was on the phone and could feel the excitement, while talking. The feeling was similar to a rush of adrenaline or sense of fear that many of us experience before we get up in front of people to talk or make a presentation or speech.

As soon as I hung up the phone, a sudden weakness came over me like a wave. Both arms felt heavy. I clutched my chest thinking, *Oh, my God. This can't be happening again.* Kurt had just come home. I could barely open the door and yell to him for help. He came running.

There was no mistake this time. I was having another heart attack. My arms hurt badly. They felt swollen and heavy as if they were dragging on the floor. At the same time, it felt like a tourniquet was binding my arm and strangling it, cutting it off my body. My chest was burning and heavy. I called the doctor on duty, but at this point, I couldn't even talk on the phone. I took two baby aspirin because that was the only aspirin I had in the cupboard, and we left for the clinic.

The clinic was a solid thirty minutes away. While we were driving, following the instructions for where to report, I knew that time was being wasted. When we arrived, the doctor was waiting for me. Every step I took toward him felt as if I was walking in slow motion. My legs could hardly move no matter how badly I wanted them to move. With Kurt's help, I finally made it to the examining table.

By this time, nearly forty minutes had flown by—precious minutes lost. When the doctor saw the EKG results, he immediately called for an ambulance. More waiting. More time lost. I was thinking that my so-called "golden hour" was passing by, and I still was in a country clinic.[3] The time for optimal intervention felt short. I was scared. Thoughts of dying here were passing through my mind.

The pain was extremely bad by this time, so the doctor said that I needed pain medication. He began to look at the veins in my forearm. His hands were sweating. *Oh my god, big red flag, sweaty hands, I bet he has not done many of these!* I knew he would be incapable of inserting the PVC without hurting me and failing several times! I said, "No, don't set it in the vein"! That didn't stop him, and he tried anyway. So, with the pain of a heart attack and the goal of getting pain relief, I was angry that he would hurt me with the needle. He finally gave up and moved from my forearm to the crease of the elbow, where phlebotomists usually draw blood.

Before he proceeded, the doctor gave me a few squirts of liquid nitroglycerine, under the tongue, which had helped to relieve the pain a little but not enough. As he inserted the needle, I could hear and feel a ripping of the vein in my arm. *Oh my god the pain in my arm!* Tears squirted out of my eyes as I begged him to stop. A lump formed immediately that was so immense I couldn't even draw my arm up. I was furious. He then gave me a shot of morphine.

Abruptly, but blessedly, the morphine kicked in. After that, I didn't care quite so much about everything. My pain was dulled, but my mind worked underneath the painkiller's fog. I remember thinking that the heart attack was *still* happening. I just was not feeling it to the same degree. *Hopefully*, I thought, *the nitro will kick in, and the blood flow will be restored.*

---

3 The "golden hour" is a term used to indicate that the sooner a person received medical treatment after a traumatic injury like a heart attack or an automobile accident, the more likely the person will survive.

Lincoln Park Library

The Hospital Stay

When I finally got to the hospital, there was more waiting, but once the medical team began working on me, they were with me every minute until I was settled into my room. A male nurse came into the room to examine my arms for placement of the PVC. He was shocked to see the needle blunders from the country clinic. When I asked him how adept he was at doing this task, he smiled and quietly said that he was exceptionally good. Happily, he was excellent. I was still having pain, so the doctors ordered more morphine, although not so much as to make me unconscious.

The phlebotomist came in and drew the blood to measure my cardiac enzymes. Meanwhile, I couldn't believe this was happening again. It had only been six weeks since I was here in this hospital with the same symptoms. The doctors were puzzled, as well. Everything looked normal by previous tests, but my symptoms were unmistakably that of a heart attack.

I finally got settled in my room, back in the five-person room with the geriatric group. *Jeez, I'm like a spring chicken compared to the older gals in the cardiac ward.* A nurse came in to hook me up to a holter monitor, which is a portable EKG/ECG or electrocardiogram device used to monitor the heart. The use of a holter monitor is known as cardiac telemetry. Fifteen minutes later, the nurse came back, wondering why there was no signal at the nurse's desk. She turned the unit over to find out there was no battery. *That's comforting!* When I'm sick, my tolerance for even minor mistakes is minimal, and that error was significant.

The doctor decided that I needed to be monitored closely, so I was moved to another room. At last, I had a private room. But my mind, which would not slow down or shut off, began to wonder whether being alone was actually such a good thing. I tried to relax, but couldn't, I was too stressed.

The next visitor was a nurse who brought a beta-blocker tablet. Thirty minutes later, I began to feel sick to my stomach and started sweating profusely or diaphoreses. I called for the nurse and asked her to open the window. The nurse quickly took an EKG. The night doctor ran in after her with her laptop to do an echocardiogram (or ECHO), which is an ultrasound of the heart. The doctor didn't say what the problem was, just that everything appeared normal. They told me to relax and brought me cold towels to ease the sweating.

I was fine until I took the beta-blocker. Something was wrong, but they were not saying anything. Well, maybe that's good for me not to know until it's something definite since I would just lay here and start thinking too much. But I was already thinking too much. I knew there was a correlation between the beta-blocker, nausea, and profuse sweating. I decided not to take that pill again. When I asked what the pill was, they refused to tell me. With everything that was happening, I felt uncertain about exactly what was happening.

It seemed that every time I closed my eyes, I suddenly found myself in the hallway walking with people that looked half-dead. Either I must be dreaming, or that morphine must still be affecting me. *It's 1:00 AM, and I'm walking with the near dead.* I buzzed the nurse and asked her to turn on the TV because I was afraid to sleep. When she asked why, I told her that every time I closed my eyes I saw dead people in the hallways. She said: "Don't worry. You are not going to die."

A Diagnosis

The next morning, a nurse greeted me and said that results from my cardiac enzyme test revealed that I had suffered another heart attack. She explained that this heart attack was seven times worse than the first, but it still fell into the mild range.

I couldn't hold back my tears; I was in disbelief and denial. *Why is this happening?* At first, I thought it was odd that a nurse delivered the results, only because it has always been my experience that the doctor explains the results, diagnosis and prognosis. Maybe this is how it is done in Norway, but I felt angry and ignored in that the doctor himself didn't come in and tell me this news. I could see him at the nurse's station with his back turned toward me. It made me think that he didn't care or that he didn't have any bedside manner or even that he was afraid or incapable of delivering distressing news. The nurse said that she could ask the doctor to come in and talk to me.

That action couldn't soothe me. Between the terrible news and the doctor's poor bedside manners, I cried out: "Why? He can't tell me any more than what you just told me!" However, at the same time, deep inside, I wanted someone with authority to tell me—it was going to be okay. Then, I couldn't stop crying. The words, *seven times worse than the first attack* kept repeating itself, in a continuous loop, over and over, *seven times worse than the first attack*. The nurse told me that she would be right back. A few minutes later, she returned and handed me sedative! What's this for? Is this how we deal with things, we get upset and take a pill? That only upset me more because the health care providers seemed to come running with such pills as soon as I began to feel any emotional discomfort. In the years since, I have spoken to other female cardiac patients who reported the same kind of treatment. When they expressed emotions, they were given tranquilizers!

More Tests

Later, a different doctor — the attending physician — came to my room and told me that he was quite interested in learning the cause of these two heart attacks since they were so close together. He suggested that I have a cardiac magnetic resonance imaging (cMRI) noninvasive study to look at my heart. However, since my cardiac enzymes were elevated, he recommended that I should have both the cMRI and another angiography. I didn't want to go through the angiography again since it was somewhat dangerous, uncomfortable, and didn't reveal anything six weeks before. I had no confidence that the test would find anything now. I felt pretty hopeless.

While I was waiting for the angiography, I was transferred from my private room to a two-person room. A new cardiologist introduced himself and told me that they were not sure why my heart attacks happened. He thought that maybe I had some type of microvascular (small artery) spasm that would not show up on the angiography. He indicated that perhaps this microvascular spasm was on a smaller branch of an artery toward the end of the heart. He recommended that I should simply go home and "wait for another heart attack" so the artery would occlude itself and become easier to detect. He said, "This is not going to kill you."

By then it was clear to me that even in the same field of study, doctors didn't look at heart disease or patients in the same ways. I didn't appreciate his suggestion and thought it was both unprofessional and genuinely bad advice. In addition, I overheard him talking with the resident doctors outside my room, telling them that health professionals like me are "stress monsters." With those careless words, he interjected a serious bias to the residents about me and undermined the potential patient doctor relationship with every one of them—including the one between him and me.

Despite overall excellent care, I was learning that individual health care providers can ruin a positive impression and lose a patient's trust quickly with poor bedside manners, bad advice, or an untoward glance at the wrong time. In fact, these providers often are found to be difficult to work with by their peers and other patients. My primary doctor told me not to give his words any importance or value whatsoever. She indicated that she didn't care for him either. In fact, one nurse said he was "special," which was meant in a derogatory way and not a compliment in the Norwegian language.

When it was time for my second angiography, I found myself again dreading the entire procedure even though I had been given tranquilizers. While I was in the hallway waiting, a fledgling doctor introduced himself: "I will be the doctor performing your angiography today." I thought he was such a young man that he had to be in his residency program. I asked him, "How many have you done?" He tilted his head and looked up at the ceiling as if to count. I thought: *Forget it!* I replied: "I am sorry. No offense to you, but you will NOT be doing it. I want the older doctor that did my first angiography, and if I cannot have him, there will be no angiography for me today." The young doctor was stunned by my words, but there was no way I was going to be his guinea-pig patient. There was hustling and bustling about in the hallway and conversations behind closed doors. Soon, the young doctor returned and told me that the other doctor would perform the angiography after he finished with another patient.

This time I asked the doctor if he could try doing the angiography from my arm instead of my groin. Unfortunately, it had to be done in the groin. Frustratingly, the second angiography again showed no significant results, which made me feel as if I had been given a healthy dose of radiation for nothing. The mystery continued.

Shortly after the procedure and while lying flat on my back, I began to feel strange—hot, sweaty, and nauseous. As I started reaching for the call button the nurse ran into my room, looked at the monitors overhead, and flipped my bed into Trendelenburg position. In this position, my feet are placed higher than my head, thereby, increasing the blood flow to my upper body. All the while, I felt as though I was slipping into a dark abyss. I couldn't open my eyes. I felt paralyzed unable to move, but my sense of hearing seemed particularly heightened and I was aware throughout the entire ordeal.

I wondered if I was dying and thought: *They say your sense of hearing is the last thing to go…very strange.* I could hear the young resident's voice, saying maybe it's a cardiac tamponade (pressure on the heart from fluid buildup in the pericardium, or sac surrounding the heart). I tried to say "no" and struggled to open my eyes, but I couldn't move. I was cognizant but paralyzed. I could just imagine him with the needle coming towards me. I wanted to stop him before he tried to stab the large needle into my chest to reduce fluid buildup.

Meanwhile, the nurses were trying to find a vein on my left side to push fluids. Although I had a central line on my right side, the echo machine was on that side, obscuring access to the line. I could hear the code being called over the loud speaker and my room number. I could hear the nurses and doctors rushing in with their crash carts, but I was past caring. It was a strange sensation to be unconscious yet fully aware of my surroundings. There wasn't a bright light to walk toward, so I was sure that I was not dying and that I would pull out of this episode soon.

Sure enough, as fast as it began, the problem ended. I asked the nurse what had happened, and she said my blood pressure had dropped to 60/20. They thought the vagus nerve had gotten over stimulated or maybe I'd just had another heart attack. Again, they didn't know.

By this time, I just wanted to go home. In the hospital, I expected to understand what was wrong. But all this not knowing was even more frustrating there than at home. I decided to get second and third opinions once I got home. I was not going to be passive and wait for the doctors to figure out what was wrong. I was tired of waiting around feeling like I was doing nothing.

Discharge Summary, Second Time Around

When I was discharged, my medical summary revealed that the ramus circumflex (intermediate coronary artery) was normal. There seemed to be possible heart wall changes at the intersection of the diagonal and marginal branches although there were no obvious changes since the angiogram six weeks prior. The right coronary artery appeared normal. The conclusion was that my heart had good left ventricular function with a few possible heart wall changes but — again — there was no significant narrowing of the arteries.

The new TnT levels revealed an elevation, which again showed a possible small non-Q infarction. Overall, the records showed the possibility of either a spasm angina caused by wall changes or a thrombosis (blood clot), which spontaneously dislodged. The doctors were challenged in part because the heart attack hadn't required their direct intervention for resolution.

The doctor recommended the same medications — particularly oral anticoagulation or blood thinning and anti-clotting drugs. He ordered additional tests to determine whether the levels of anti-clotting drugs were sufficient. We discussed the new course of medication. The doctor suggested that I should have a beta blocker. I reminded him of what happened the last time I took a beta blocker, and that I was reluctant to try it again. We compromised with a calcium channel blocker, Norvasc (amlodipine) instead. He wanted me to use it to address the possibility of spasm angina, which I might have been experiencing. He also prescribed a nitroglycerine (nitro) spray for use by mouth in emergency situations.

The Third Heart Attack

The adage about bad things happening in threes seems to be true. Exactly a month after my second heart attack, I had a third one.

My husband, Kurt and I were walking on the back trails of an old railroad station near Hellvik. It was a beautiful Sunday walk, fairly flat as railroad trails tend to be. On the way back, shortly after we had turned around, I noticed that Kurt kept getting farther and farther away. I was having trouble keeping up. I wondered why he was going so fast, but it was me, I suddenly felt breathless and extremely fatigued. Every step I took was so incredibly tiring that I felt I could not take one more step. I stopped cold in my tracks. Kurt noticed that I was no longer beside him and he turned around and walked back. Concerned, he asked, "What's wrong?" I replied, "I cannot walk any farther." Kurt suggested that I sit down. Then, I started feeling indigestion. Thinking this indigestion could have been from my lunch, I just sat on the side of the trail burping.

New to this game, I was internally justifying that I could not be having another heart attack by calling the sensation "indigestion." In hindsight, I should have taken the nitro spray prescribed by my doctor. At worst I would have gotten a headache from the dose, which is a small price to pay. Kurt checked his mobile phone and wanted to call the ambulance, but I begged him not to. I didn't want to go back into the hospital. Even if I hadn't been so stubborn, he had no cell signal where we were walking. Kurt was panicking because I couldn't take another step. We were alone on the trail, and he had no way to call for help. Even now, despite my stronger heart, we know we will never again walk in that remote place or in any place without cell signal.

All of a sudden, after a little more than a half hour, I regained my strength and was able to walk. Later that day, my mind cleared, and I realized that I had all the symptoms of another heart attack — this time without the pain. But was that a heart attack? Is this called a silent heart attack that can occur without pain? I felt only indigestion and overwhelming fatigue, not tightness in the chest or arms like I did with the second heart attack.

I called my doctor first thing Monday morning and was told to have blood drawn for a troponin test. My doctor called with the results as soon as she got them; my troponin was elevated, suggesting I had another heart attack, but it was one number from the clinically accepted level for a heart attack. A tiny number difference would have put me in the hospital for the third time.

So the news was bittersweet: no hospital stay with its pokes, prods, and indignities, but another heart attack with the undeniable knowledge that I wasn't out of the woods yet. Since 2005, troponin tests have been made even more sensitive, which means that this third heart attack likely would have called for another hospitalization.

That night, I woke up in a panic with a feeling of unrest and sudden doom. I tried to blow it off and relax. I was in bed resting, after all. I thought the feeling would just go away if I lay down and went back to sleep. Twenty minutes later, I woke up again, scared to death for no apparent reason. My heart pounded like it was trying to jump out of my chest. I got out of bed because I had started belching.

It was 2:00 AM, and I was looking at my nitro spray. *Should I take it, or shouldn't I?* Back and forth I went, asking *should I or shouldn't I?* I wasn't sure because I couldn't recall any health care professional telling me exactly when I should take it. Online, I had found a reputable site that indicated when and how to use the nitro spray; but lacking my doctor's instructions, I felt unsure. I decided to opt for the potential headache over the likelihood of another heart attack.

Within a few minutes, I felt relief from both indigestion burps and the heart pounding that gave me a sense of having a knife in my back. After this night, I knew that if I had any doubt at all about my symptoms, I should not hesitate to reach for the nitro. For a year after my heart attacks, I took it as soon as possible. The key, I learned, is prevention. Don't be afraid to take your nitro.

The headache I got from it was mild and felt more like a flushing and pulsing in the back of my head. These sensations were nothing compared to the sense of relief I felt. I learned to take the nitro if there was any doubt in my mind.

Why was taking the nitro such a big deal for me? I don't like taking medications to begin with, and I was on a number of prescribed drugs at that time. Adding the nitro was one more medication requirement that went against my fundamental desire not to use drugs. But the main reason I didn't want to take the nitro was more of an internal struggle; by using that medication, I was admitting, *Yes, I'm a heart patient.*

This feeling of being less than healthy and having a real medical problem was a slippery slope, and it could be very dangerous. If I denied reality and didn't take the medication, I could potentially die. If I took the medication, then the reality of being a heart patient crashed into me.

There was one more issue; however, that was fundamental in keeping me from taking the medication: no one ever explained when to take it. I knew how to take it—under the tongue. The big issue for me was differentiating between indigestion and possible heart attack. I didn't want to take the medication if I was simply having indigestion. For women, this is a big issue as heart attacks seem to present in this manner.

So, I stopped eating all things that might cause indigestion. In my case those foods were tomatoes, onions, and garlic—but these differ for everyone. By eliminating the gas-causing foods, I found I could make a better decision about whether my heart was experiencing a problem.

However, it isn't wise to make decisions about taking nitro, an important first-response medication, based only on food choices. We need to be much more assertive when prescribed such a medication and (1) ask the doctor why the drug is being prescribed and how to use it and understand the criteria for its use (2) ask the pharmacist for more information about it.

The 2012 guidelines from the College of Cardiology Foundation/American Heart Association Task Force on Angina/Non-ST Elevation Myocardial Infarction state the following:

"If patients experience chest discomfort/pain and have been previously prescribed NTG (nitroglycerine) and have it available, it's recommended that they be instructed (in advance) to take 1 dose of NTG immediately in response to symptoms. If chest discomfort/pain is unimproved or worsening 5 minutes after taking 1 NTG sublingually, it's recommended that the patient call 9-1-1 immediately.

In patients with chronic stable angina, if the symptoms are significantly improved after taking 1 NTG, it's appropriate to instruct the patient or family member/friend/caregiver to repeat NTG every 5 minutes for a maximum of 3 doses and call 9-1-1 if symptoms have not totally resolved." (Wright et al., 2010)

Getting the right information and following the instructions for nitro and other cardio assistive medications can be vital to survival, so be assertive and find out what to do as soon as the medicine is prescribed.

One final suggestion is necessary here. It's often possible to find a cardiac rehabilitation (cardiac rehab) unit where you can get help in the initial recovery phases from a heart attack. While I couldn't find one near my home in Norway, I was most interested in cardiac rehab because I could be monitored there and feel safe about doing anything physical. Ask your doctor about the benefits of cardiac rehab for your recovery process.

Lessons Learned

1. My second heart attack presented with entirely different symptoms. I knew instantly I was having a heart attack, and I immediately took two aspirins. After the second heart attack, I now have effervescent aspirin in my medicine cabinet. My new symptoms were:

   a) Pain in the chest.

   b) A burning and heavy sensation.

   c) Pain down the left arm and feeling like a tourniquet binding and strangling the arm.

2. If doctors are unsure of whether you have had a heart attack because of unusual or mild symptoms, ask for the cardiac enzymes test. The TnT test is sensitive enough to reveal damage from even a mild heart attack.

3. Be prepared for additional tests and ongoing investigation into your heart attack. Possible tests include:

   a) Blood tests

   b) Cardiac MRIs

   c) Angiograms

4. Cardioprotective medication may be needed.

   a) Aspirin. Since I had prior experience from the first heart attack, I knew that I needed to take aspirin right away. Talk to your doctor about different varieties of aspirin and keep it handy for emergency use as recommended by your doctor.

   b) Prescription blood thinning medications.

c) Anti-clotting drugs.

d) Cholesterol drugs.

e) Nitroglycerine. If you have had a confirmed heart attack, ask about a prescription for nitro tablet, spray, or transdermal patches. Make sure you know how and when to take it.

5. Have someone you trust with you when discharged and when medications are prescribed. This person should ask any questions that you might not think of, and he or she should pay particular attention to when, why, and how to take those medications.

THREE
CHAPTER

One Man's Heart

My understanding of heart disease originally came from watching my father struggle with his heart health. At the time, my best friend was a cardiac nurse, and she gave me an introduction to cardiac health. At first, I was an observer, and eventually I became his advocate as his health deteriorated and he needed a heart transplant. This account of my father's heart condition won't pertain to everyone. However, what I learned from my father's history informed my responses to my own heart attacks, as I described them in Chapters One and Two. In this chapter, I introduce some more heart-specific terminology and some of the choices that Dad needed to make more than thirty years ago.

My Father's Heart

Many women only know about the symptoms of the male pattern of heart disease, thinking that all heart attacks present with crushing chest pain that radiates to the left arm. However, many people experience symptoms similar to indigestion, ignore those symptoms, and deny that anything serious is wrong. Although I have struggled with belief and disbelief about my heart condition, my doctors here in Norway were surprised I made it to the hospital for help as quickly as I did. I got help rapidly because I listen to my body. In the U. S., I also was a certified emergency medical technician-defibrillator (EMT 1A-D), certified in basic (BCLS) and advanced cardiac life support (ACLS). These trainings helped me to recognize symptoms of illness although I didn't consciously connect them to heart disease.

Just as important to my own heart health, my father became a heart patient when I was seventeen years old. In the 1970s, less was known about how to heal the heart and heart patients with my father's problems didn't have many surgical options. Most doctors learned to manage cardiac patients with medications. Dad was on medication for at least ten years before he started to deteriorate. I watched him suffer tremendously over the years. It sounds cynical, but I came to believe that because hospital administrations are interested in surgical statistics from both a reputation and financial standpoint, if they think a patient might not survive a surgery, then he or she is less likely to be considered a candidate. From my perspective, this situation seemed true in my father's case.

Dad's Illness

My father suffered a major heart attack on my seventeenth birthday. I remember that night clearly, he was belching and sweating profusely. Dad told me he had indigestion, and he certainly didn't look well. He assured me that he would be okay. The next morning, my mother woke me up and said she was taking Dad to the hospital. It was touch and go for the first forty-eight hours. The doctors said that my dad had suffered a major MI (heart attack) to the left ventricle and the next twenty-four hours would determine his prognosis.

For many years, Dad stayed with his doctor and didn't seek a second opinion. He believed he was in capable hands and had excellent care. After ten years of medication for his ischemia (a condition where the heart doesn't receive enough blood), the medicine was no longer working. At that point, my father began to question his doctor about having a coronary artery bypass graft (CABG). The doctor said he wasn't a surgical candidate because he believed my father would die on the table. After that news, Dad was skeptical about getting a second opinion.

In retrospect, my father regretted not getting a second and third opinion. He believed that if he had been proactive much sooner and had a CABG, he never would have needed the transplant he later received. Dad's situation is why I didn't wait to seek alternative treatments when I had my heart attacks. In fact, one day after school, my youngest daughter Kirsten said, "Hey mom, why don't you check out stem cells for your heart." *Stem cells, huh.* This was the beginning of my new journey in life, which you will find out later in Chapter 10.

On Dad's behalf, I began a quest to find a more progressive, forward thinking doctor. Once found, the new doctor immediately scheduled Dad for quintuple bypass surgery within two weeks. Dad was taken aback because he had two different doctors with diametric approaches on how to treat his condition. I told him that we could get a third opinion to help him decide; however, he chose to accept the progressive doctor's approach as he started to become refractory to the medications.

The damage to his heart was substantial, and there was a sac filled with clots hanging from the apex of his heart. The surgeons needed to find a line of demarcation and cut the injured part away, which left him with two thirds of a heart. Recent medical research tells us that the elliptical shape of the heart is crucial, and surgeons now know not to cut away the apex of the heart.

For two years, Dad did exceptionally. His only medication was one aspirin a day. He felt healthy again and wished he would have had the surgery sooner since the damage to his heart and the scar tissue had been massive. After two short years, however, my father suddenly began to feel weak. He went back to the hospital and had a pacemaker implanted, but it lasted only two years before it couldn't help him anymore. By then, my father was in such poor shape that he had to be put on the heart transplant list.

The Transplant

I started to research all I could find about heart transplants, which was much less information in the mid-1980s than now. I was doing research the old fashioned way; there were no computers like today. I visited all the biomedical libraries I could find in southern California. Armed with medical abstracts and clinical studies, I went to my father's house and explained the pros and cons of the procedure. Simply put, without the transplant, he would die; however, with the transplant, there was a chance—not a certainty—that he could live longer. My father's response was: "You're a good salesperson, Dori." Of course, I was just giving him the facts as they were at that time, and Dad opted for the transplant. The possibility of life over the certainty of death is what actually persuaded my father.

The next steps involved more research. We needed to find out which doctors had the greatest success and lowest mortality rate. Next, we needed to interview the potential doctors and discuss the logistics of the surgery. My father asked, "Shouldn't my doctors be doing what you are doing?" Thinking that I would be putting more attention to the process than busy doctors, I told him that I was happy to do the research and investigative work. His primary cardiologist thanked me for my efforts. The research was, in fact, his job.

However, with great attention to detail, I coordinated the whole process and was the liaison between the transplant team and Dad's cardiologist. From an early age, I have thought it's important to have an advocate to help with complex medical visits and decision making. I was Dad's advocate.

We found a great hospital for his transplant. Then, after all other arrangements were made, we simply had to wait. After some time on the transplant list, the doctors told us that my father had about two weeks left to live. I felt so sad and sorry for him. What could I say to my father? The idea that he had only two weeks left to live seared my own heart. I thought: *He must know he is dying. He looks like a skeleton with skin – he is so skinny. He's scared, afraid of dying, dreaming of white sheets, and afraid to go to sleep.*

Sometimes when I was home, I sensed I could see him out of the corner of my eye sitting in his favorite chair. It gave me chills. I wondered what I should say to him. I wanted to say something that had meaning beyond simple greetings and idle talk. There was no time left for meaningless noise that would simply fill the dead space and waste precious moments. No, I wanted to say something more, but what could I say?

For three days, all I could think about was my father and what I could say to him. Every night, I would pray the same thing and ask God to give me the words to fill my father's tired heart with hope and peace. I would ask, *God, please give me the words for my Dad*. One night, God gave me those words in a profound dream—or vision, as some may call it. I couldn't fathom the depths of the peace and serenity that it gave to me. The next day, I couldn't wait to get to the hospital to tell my father the good news that he didn't have to be afraid of death.

My Dream

On the night of my transcendent experience, my thoughts for the past three days and nights had been consumed by thoughts of my father. Dad used to tell me stories of how his father raised him in India with Hindu beliefs. Since he married my mother and she was Catholic, he converted. I wondered what it was like for my dad having experienced these two very distinct belief systems.

Frankly, I didn't know what he believed at this point. Did he believe in reincarnation or an afterlife? As a child and teenager, we never spoke about deep spiritual issues but about the practicalities of life. However, I was fascinated about different beliefs and took all the high school and college classes that I could take about different religions. In high school, I signed up for a class based on the Elizabeth Kúbler Ross' book, *On Death and Dying*. There were only five students in the class.

I think I took that class as a way to cope with the death of a young adult friend who had died suddenly in my arms from an asthma attack that went into full cardiac arrest. I'm reminded often of what I learned there as my life unfolds. At the time, I wondered why it was necessary for a sixteen-year old to have an understanding of the challenges of coming to grips with one's upcoming death. By the time I was seventeen, I knew. My father had his first heart attack.

Years later, as I lay in bed pondering my father's need for a heart and his possible death, I prayed with intent and focus: *God, put the words in my mouth. Give me something meaningful to say to my father.* One night my prayers were answered, and I was awakened by a loud, thundering clap. I woke up! I was scared. I heard a deeply resonant voice say: *Wake up. I have something to show you.*

I remember stepping out of bed and looking at my feet; they were those of a child. I was a little girl. I looked up and saw a tall angelic man with wings. He protectively spread a wing over me, and we walked. He told me not to be afraid, and that everything would be alright. Although we were not talking with our mouths, I could hear him clearly in my head.

We walked in the clouds, up, and up — the path seemed to go on forever. Then, suddenly, we stopped. He said, *Behold!* And he took his wing off me. I looked up, and the light that was shining was so beautiful that I still cannot describe it with words other than to say it was ineffable. "Magnificent" cannot do justice to that light. Behind the light, I could see a figure of man and the silhouette of a heart, but the light was blindingly intense, and I knew that I could not gaze directly upon what I was seeing. I felt as though my eyes would catch on fire, so I looked away.

I felt a deep sense of reverence as I dropped to my knees and proclaimed in wonder: *Oh my god! There really is a God!* I put my hands up to feel the presence of the light. And for the first time in my life, I felt complete and unconditional love. Every cell in my body was being pumped full of Love from the light. It was incredible. For the first time I now understand real Love. It is beyond anything I have ever experienced!

The angelic man told me that it was time to go back. When I said, *No, I like it here,* he said, *you have to hurry.* There were no words exchanged. We simply spoke again with our minds. As he and I walked back to where we had begun, I saw some figures like silhouettes of people who were warm and seemed to welcome me to stay. I realized that on some level, they recognized me, and I felt a connection, too. Although I didn't know any of them, somehow my spirit recognized them. Suddenly, I realized that humans are all the same inside. We are all connected as spiritual brothers and sisters.

During these moments, I was rationalizing that it was fine to stay in this beautiful, supernatural place and that Kurt could take care of our (then) two children. Later, it seemed profound that I was entirely willing to walk away from a family that I can't consciously conceive of abandoning.

The angelic man brought me back down to my bed. I remember lying down, and as soon as I did, I was wide awake. I said again to myself: *There really is a God!* Before this experience, I had known love. But, I had not realized what a greater Love can feel like. As humans, we have no idea that our capacity to love is so incredibly immense. My sense of that Love was of being complete beyond the love I felt for my spouse, my children, or anyone else I had ever loved. This feeling, I believe, is Love on a cellular level.

After this vision, my spirit was filled with peace and unequivocally no fear of death. I knew this was the message I was to give to my father. I had begged for the words to speak to my father, and here they were.

That day, I could not wait to tell Dad about my dream. When I told him, he wondered whether I had a near-death experience. I said: "No, I had a vision. It came to me during my sleep. I remember it perfectly, and it was a message for you." He became peaceful and didn't seem afraid anymore.

Remarkably, a heart became available within those two crucial weeks.

Life after the Transplant

Dad went through the transplant and survived the surgery despite some tough odds. I remember that the operation was an exceedingly long procedure. As my father's primary advocate, I was elected the spokesperson for the family, which spared my poor mother the challenges of navigating the medical jungle. She was, of course, emotionally shredded over the whole ordeal. The team was wonderful — caring, compassionate, and excellent communicators. This was the finest medical team I have ever and since met. They worked together for my father the way doctors should work when it comes to both medical skill and communication. They were phenomenal.

After the transplant, my father believed that all the waiting and pain and anxiety were worthwhile.

For readers considering a heart transplant, let me explain briefly about my father's quality of life from the caregiver's perspective. After Dad had the transplant surgery, while he was in the hospital recovering, he developed the cytomegalovirus virus or CMV, which resulted in over fifty esophageal ulcers. During that illness, he was hemorrhaging and in terrible pain. In fact, he said that experience was worse than the transplant surgery and recovery.

A transplant patient must be on immunosuppressive drugs that help to prevent rejection of the received organ. This drug therapy continues for the entire lifetime of the patient. Having immunosuppressive therapy, suppresses the immune system this means that if the patient comes into contact with someone who has a cold, the germs could easily infect the patient's body and quickly morph into a more serious illness like pneumonia. To stay well, Dad usually wore a mask when he went out in public and always around small children, who carry many germs in their little bodies.

Because of all the steroids he was prescribed, Dad's hips severely degraded. He not only had two hip replacements, but even those hip replacements couldn't work perfectly and they dislocated several times. When his hips were dislocated on two separate occasions, he was not allowed to go to the Memorial Hospital ten minutes away in Long Beach to his home cardiologist. Instead, because Dad had the heart transplant done in San Diego, he had to go there for treatment. The result was that he had to endure more than two hours in the ambulance with a dislocated hip.

As Dad's heart health became more precarious, the doctors told him that he couldn't have another transplant because his bones were too brittle from all the drugs. He was on so much prednisone, a corticosteroid that suppresses the immune system that he developed a moonlike face: his face became round like a ball and nearly twice the size. My youngest daughter became afraid of him and wouldn't go to him although the older children knew his face well enough to recognize him as their loving grandfather. Sadly, Dad had more sick days than well days, but to him the entire transplant process was worth the challenges it presented. There are some lucky ones that make it without complication but not my father.

My father died five years after transplant. The doctors were stumped. There was no clear reason for his decline as he had been doing well. Some type of trigger went off in his body, and he began producing cholesterol at levels drugs could not control. Frighteningly, the ischemia that took his first heart was now claiming his second. No matter what kind or how much medication the doctors gave him, nothing worked. It was devastating to see my father so full of hope with his renewed life and having that life changed again.

On July 22, 1992, I got the call from my mother that my father had died at the age of sixty-three. She said to hurry, and the hospital would keep his body for me. When I arrived, Dad was lying in a room by himself with the curtains drawn shut. He looked so peaceful and tranquil. I leaned over, caressed his face, and told him that now he could finally be at peace. The nurse who was with him when he died told me that he was remarkably calm in his last moments. I'm glad he was not alone.

Oddly, my father's survival time may be linked to a conversation he had with his doctor. Shortly after the transplant, Dad, a scientist and aerospace engineer, asked, "How long do I have with the new heart?" The doctor replied, "Statistically, 80% don't make it past five years." And nearly five years to the day, my father died. Sometimes I think he became his own self-fulfilling prophecy as if he had given himself exactly five years to live. I sometimes wonder whether Dad might have survived longer if he had been told that the 80% survival rate was ten years. As I explain in later chapters, I believe the mind has a lot of power over our bodies.

My father's experience makes me believe that it's crucial not to listen to negative statistics about our medical conditions. Much of our health is connected to the mind and the spirit. The body/mind/spirit connection has been well studied and demonstrated scientifically. Negative statistics get sucked into our thoughts, and we tend to believe them. The power of belief is great—especially when an authority figure like a doctor tells us something. When we are sick our minds are extremely vulnerable and open to suggestions.

It's critical not to get caught up in the numbers that represent other people's experiences. Remember that it is only a segment of the population. We are all unique human beings; what one person experiences is not another's experience. The doctors are not gods, either. They are human like the rest of us. As my experiences with my second heart attack showed very clearly, doctors don't have all the answers. We need to keep in mind that the human body is an amazing creation and the mind and spirit are even more incredible.

Lessons Learned

1. In the 1970s and 1980s, there were fewer options for men (or women) with various kinds of heart disease. Both

medical and surgical options were limited. There are more choices for heart patients than my father had, so be open to doctors' suggestions at the same time as being responsible for researching them and getting second and even third opinions.

2. Even good or reasonable medical choices have consequences. For my father, a quintuple bypass surgery was performed, and because his heart damage was substantial, one third of his heart was cut away — leading to a nonelliptical shape of the heart that doctors now know is not ideal. It's important to know that medical science will continue to develop knowledge and procedures; therefore, the surgery my father had — and its risks — have to be understood in the context of the time it was done. A transplant is one option for some heart patients, but it's an option with lifelong consequences for general health and the need for ongoing medication. The immunosuppressive medication has serious consequences. If at all possible, opt for whatever healing measures you can before a transplant is considered necessary. For example, I had one patient that wanted stem cell treatment. She was on a transplant list. All she wanted to do was pick up her grandson and walk up the stairs. But she wanted the choice to try stem cells in an effort to save her heart, and if it didn't work, she would be back on the transplant list. She came for treatment and, as a result, after five years, she is doing remarkable well with her ejection fraction in the normal range. Realize that stem cell treatment is not an option for everyone. However, if you are refractory to medical treatment and you are a no option patient it may be worth investigating. I know if my dad were alive today, I would have undoubtedly urged him to try stem cells before transplant. Once you have a transplant, that's it there is no turning back. I

have worked with several physicians and their patient's seeking stem cell treatment.

3. Research, research, research. Go into any surgical or medical procedure as an informed patient.

4. Get second and third opinions. That's what doctors are paid to do. They don't mind. Responsible doctors want you to make choices that are best for you. We would ask my father's doctors, "Would this be something you would recommend to your father or mother?" Thirty-five years ago, they seemed shocked that we would ask this question, but it gave them a different perspective and some would change their recommendation.

5. Heart health requires positive thinking. It's easy to let poor statistics influence your thinking about your health potential. Try to remember that the numbers represent a small segment of the population and other people's experiences. You can co-create your own experiences with your own thinking and beliefs.

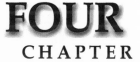

FOUR

CHAPTER

A Woman's Heart

My research into heart disease has led me to understand that women present different symptoms than men, and they express their experiences differently, too. Women also tend to be treated differently than men in the hospital, and they have had different treatment in research studies historically. Women's symptoms often are somewhat vague or are expressed in a way that some doctors haven't heard before. Sometimes, doctors dismiss the female patient as one who is experiencing an emotional or psychological problem rather than a physical one.

I wonder how many women have paid the ultimate price with their life. Many women don't recognize the symptoms of a heart attack and many doctors don't understand the difference between female and male heart patterns for an MI. This chapter explains some of the risks that are specific to women with the goal of helping us to communicate better with the medical community.

Women, This Is Not Your Father's Heart Disease

I refused to believe that I was predestined to suffer the same fate as my father. Please don't misunderstand what I'm saying. It's possible to have a family predisposition for heart disease, such as familial cardiomyopathy, caused by a defective gene. At the same time, one can have heart disease histories from both sides of the family, which increases the likelihood of heart disease. In my father's case, no one knew of any familial predispositions to heart disease, but they could have existed. Nonetheless, his lifestyle—smoking, eating too much, unresolved anger issues, and a high pressure job—was conducive to poor heart health. My father also ignored the signs of impending heart disease.

Although anyone can make poor lifestyle choices that may lead to heart disease, there are genuine physical differences between men and women. As I started to investigate my own heart attacks, I found some clear distinctions between the sexes.

Heart disease is no longer considered a man's problem. In fact, it's the leading cause of death in women in the U. S. According to the American Heart Association, 60% of all heart attacks occur in women. In 2010, it was estimated that 785,000 of that 60% would suffer a recurring heart attack. Nearly every minute, a woman dies from heart disease. Indeed, according to the Yale medical library: "Of the approximately 500,000 fatal heart attacks per year, almost half occur in women. Women who have a heart attack are twice as likely to die within the first two weeks as are men" (Rosenfeld, 1992). In the U. S. alone, there are more than 42 million women that have heart disease (Roger et al., 2011). Worldwide, nearly 8.6 million women die every year from cardiovascular diseases (WHO, 2003).

Unfortunately, sometimes people think that heart disease only happens in older women because they are no longer protected by their hormones. However, heart disease hits younger women at incredibly high rates. It's the third cause of death among women ages twenty-five to forty-four, and it's the second cause of death for women ages forty-five to sixty-four years (CDC, 2007). Many people would be surprised by these statistics because women's heart disease has not received the same kind of media attention as breast cancer, for example, as a threat to women's lives.

Women are not the only ones who don't know enough about women's cardiovascular disease. In a 2005, an American Heart Association study showed that only 8% of primary care physicians and 17% of cardiologists knew that heart disease kills more women than men. Today is not that much different. In fact, 90% of primary care doctors don't know that heart disease kills more women than men, according to the American Heart Association (Mosca et al., 2005).

Gender Bias
Gender Bias in Studies

Given the widespread belief that heart disease is a man's disease, the majority of cardiovascular research has excluded women. This failure to study women is a blatant example of gender bias. As much as three quarters of clinical studies evaluating therapies for treating heart failure through the 1980s and 1990s were conducted with men as the subjects. Women comprised only 24% of participants in all heart-related studies.

The common belief once was that when women reach meno-pause, our risk of developing a heart attack or coronary heart disease (CHD) becomes the same as a man's.[4] Little was said about young or middle-aged women from ages 45-54 having heart attacks. The belief has been widespread that women have the same risks as a man after we enter our 60s. Now, however, research shows that this is not true. In fact, because it has become understood that younger women do suffer heart disease, research must now reevaluate treatment protocols. Because of the gender bias in developing treatments, medical scientists now understand that treatments based on men's bodies and ages don't work on women the same way. Treatments developed for men may not be effective for women.

In fact, researchers now recognize additional bias concerning ethnicity. African-American, Hispanic-American, and Latin-American women appear to be at a greater risk for developing heart disease compared to Caucasian women of similar socioeconomic status (American Heart Association, 2006). Therefore, not only are more women's focused studies needed, but also studies regarding ethnic backgrounds in women.

Why have women been excluded from most studies thus far? One reason is that women of childbearing years were excluded from clinical studies due to a federal mandate to protect women and their future offspring from potentially hazardous treatment protocols. However, with changing times and ways of thinking, the National Institutes of Health now mandates that women must be included in the studies.

To further complicate matters, when it became apparent that women also suffered from CHD, treatment protocols were substandard compared to those developed for men. As a result—primarily of disbelief that women would suffer heart

---

4 Coronary heart disease (CHD) is a narrowing of the small blood vessels that supply blood and oxygen to the heart. CHD is also called coronary artery disease—or CAD—which is the most common type of heart disease.

attacks — women were four times more likely than men to receive a psychiatric diagnosis to explain CHD symptoms. On the other hand, standard treatment for men was to treat them early with immediate aspirin therapy on suspicion of a heart problem, beta-blockers, reperfusion therapy to restore blood flow, and/or urgent angioplasty. These protocols often are delayed or used to a lesser extent for women overall (Women and Heart Disease).

Gender Differences in Mortality

Fully 64% of women (versus 50% of men) who die suddenly from CHD didn't have classic warning symptoms (American Heart Association, 2006). Remember that those "classic" warning signs were derived from studies that primarily involved men, which means that these signs more often describe the male experience of a heart attack. Women often have cardiovascular symptoms that are not specific to chest pain. Two-thirds of women who die suddenly of CHD have no symptoms, probably reflecting a distinct microvasculature cause of cardiovascular disease in women (Lancet, 2011).

Under the age of fifty, in fact, women's heart attacks are twice as likely as men's to be fatal within the first few weeks after the heart attack. Moreover, 38% of women (versus 25% of men) die within one year following an MI (American Heart Association, 2006).

The statistics are shocking. Women are twice as likely as men to have heart failure, one-and-a-half times more likely to die within a year of a heart attack, and twice as likely to have a poor outcome after a coronary artery bypass graft. Furthermore, the cardiovascular mortality rate is rising in women younger than fifty-five years (Lancet, 2011).

For women, it's important to understand these differences in mortality rates. It may not necessarily be that women's heart attacks are worse than men's. Most likely, the gender bias in heart research is responsible for a higher risk of missing the heart attack in the first place and treating it unsuccessfully in the second place. This next section on risk factors for women and heart attacks should be read with care.

Gender Differences in Early Warning Signs

Knowing the early warning signs of heart attack is critical. There are vital gender differences in the body's early warnings that a heart attack may occur or is occurring.

Researchers suggest that women can have early warning signs for about a month prior to a heart attack. Women most often use these descriptions: fatigue, sleep disorders, aching, tightness, burning, pressure, and a strong sense of doom. More than 90% of women who had heart attacks reported them. Unfortunately, their symptoms were underrated, misdiagnosed, or disregarded, which led them to seek medical attention several times before proper diagnosis.

The most frequent early warning signs reported are:

1. Fatigue
2. Sleep disturbance
3. Shortness of breath
4. Indigestion
5. Increased anxiety

There may be a physiological reason that heart attacks often are mistaken for indigestion. The heart, esophagus, and stomach are in close proximity and share the vagus nerve. The stress of a heart attack appears to affect the blood flow in the stomach, and sharing that common nerve may cause the symptoms of indigestion and heart attack to appear together.

Nearly half the women studied by McSweeny et al. (2003) rated their fatigue and sleep disturbance as severe. Most women reported to have at least one early warning sign as early as one month — either daily or several times a week — before the initial onset of the acute MI. In my case, I totally overlooked these symptoms because of the whooping cough. Since my doctor had told me that I would cough for at least three months, I tended to ignore other physical sensations as being part of that problem. For example, my chest would hurt after a coughing spell, so it didn't signify anything out of the ordinary for me during that time period. In hindsight, I do remember having (and ignoring) many of the above symptoms prior to my first heart attack.

Doctors are faced with a difficult task in diagnosing women due to variations in descriptors. For example, a surprising 29.7% of women reported chest discomfort, which they described as aching, tightness, pressure, sharpness, fullness, and tingling. On the other hand, some women having a heart attack expressed that they have no symptoms, according to McSweeny et al. (2003).

You will be asked additional questions if you go to the hospital complaining of the following symptoms:

- ❤ Chest pain, pressure, tightness, or heaviness; pain that radiates to neck, jaw, shoulders, back, or to one or both arms

- ❤ Indigestion, "heartburn," nausea, and/or vomiting associated with chest discomfort

- ❤ Persistent shortness of breath

- ❤ Weakness, dizziness, lightheadedness, loss of consciousness

With these symptoms, a triage nurse will decide whether the symptoms meet the protocol of a heart attack:

- ❤ Chest pain or severe epigastric pain, non traumatic in origin, with components typical of myocardial ischemia or MI:

- ❤ Central/substernal compression or crushing chest pain

- ❤ Pressure, tightness, heaviness, cramping, burning, or aching sensation

- ❤ Unexplained indigestion, belching, or epigastric pain. Epigastric pain would be located in the center, just below the xiphoid process, between the ribs and above the umbilical. (This is also the location where you would perform the Heimlich maneuver.)

- ❤ Radiating pain in the neck, jaw, shoulders, back, or one or both arms

- ❤ Associated dyspnea (shortness of breath)

- ❤ Associated nausea and/or vomiting

- ❤ Associated diaphoresis (excessive sweating associated with shock)

If your symptoms meet the protocol, you most likely will be given a 12-lead electrocardiogram according to 2011 ACCF/AHA guidelines.

Gender Differences in Risk Factors

Both men and women must consider individual risk factors for CHD such as heredity, age, race, blood pressure, blood cholesterol, and smoking. Certain risk factors such as smoking and diabetes are more prevalent in women than men.

Heart Attack Risk Factors

Risk Factor—High Blood Pressure and Women

Nearly one-third of the American population has high blood pressure or hypertension, which is a significant risk factor for heart attack and stroke for both men and women. The increase in pressure damages the arteries. However, women have a higher risk for high blood pressure than men. Factors that contribute to high blood pressure are genetics, age, gender, menopause, and lifestyle.

If you have a family history of high blood pressure, you should have your blood pressure checked periodically. My mother's uncle died at a young age with high blood pressure and kidney failure. I never actually thought about blood pressure as a young woman. I always had low to-normal pressure until I became pregnant. After my first pregnancy, I was vigilant about taking my pressure. In fact, today, researchers now speculate that hypertension during pregnancy is a new indicator for heart problems later in life. Suddenly, in my mid-30s, I was diagnosed with high blood pressure. Today my pressure is perfect, using the practices, I outline in this book.

To understand your body's blood pressure patterns, it's helpful for you to learn how to take your own pressure. When we are newly diagnosed with high blood pressure, it's easy to be nervous in the doctor's office, which can increase or otherwise change blood pressure. This occurrence is known as "white coat syndrome," named for the doctor's white coat. I decided to desensitize myself to it because I would get two vastly different readings from home and when I would see the doctor. To overcome this kind of nervousness, I took my blood pressure and charted it several times a day. I have continued this desensitization practice for years.

Tips for taking your blood pressure include:

- ❤ Keep your arm at 90 degrees with your heart. If your arm is held too high, your pressure will register as low, and if your arm is held too low, your pressure will register as high.

- ❤ Practice taking blood pressure in both arms to chart possible differences.

- ❤ Empty your bladder before taking your blood pressure.

- ❤ Do not cross your legs or arms and do not talk while taking your blood pressure.

Lifestyle choices such as smoking, poor diet, and lack of exercise can negatively affect blood pressure. For example, a sedentary lifestyle increases chances for high blood pressure and weight gain. This is yet another reason to get into the habit of physical activity. Exercise is so crucial to our good health that it needs to become a routine like brushing our teeth. Your body was meant to move.

Similarly, a sodium-heavy diet can raise blood pressure. Where salt goes, water follows, which means fluid retention. These fluids put stress on the heart. A great deal of sodium is found in most canned, bottled, and otherwise processed foods. To lower high blood pressure, learn to make healthy food choices.

Some blood pressure problems are genetic and need medication for treatment, while other problems often can be resolved with lifestyle changes. Give the doctor a detailed family history to help in making this distinction. My doctor said that we should not feel any different when taking medication for high blood pressure. I needed to try different brands before finding the right one, though. One of the medications caused me to have a dry, hacking cough, which was a side effect. It's important to work with your doctor to get the right blood pressure medication.

Risk Factor—Smoking and Women

We know that smoking is a major risk factor for heart attacks. Smoking strips women of their cardioprotective factors of estrogen and high-density lipoprotein (HDL). Estrogen guards against heart attacks in women by increasing HDL. HDL is needed to carry out low-density lipoprotein (LDL) or the so-called "bad" cholesterol, thus preventing blockages in the arteries.

If you smoke, even if it's only one or two cigarettes a day, STOP! STOP NOW! Your life depends on it. It's easy to believe that smoking just a little (one to four cigarettes per day), instead of a whole pack, is safe. Some women justify smoking by saying: "I only smoke one or two a day; it's like not smoking at all." That's how I justified my smoking—even after my first heart attack. I only smoked one cigarette a day, so I thought it was okay. This thinking is absolutely wrong! The day that I had the second heart attack was the last time I ever smoked. I was a non-smoker when I moved to Norway; it was very much a drinking and smoking culture in social settings. I was called an "American snob" since I did not do either. So I picked up the nasty habit feeling a bit of peer pressure from my colleagues. Pathetic, I know. However, I am a non-smoker once again!

The number of cigarettes one smokes *absolutely* is associated with risk of fatal CHD, non-fatal heart attacks, and angina pectoris (chest pain, or ischemia due to blood flow) according to the Nurses' Health Study. This study states that smoking one-to-four cigarettes per day doubles a woman's risk of fatal and nonfatal CHD. Smoking five-to-fourteen cigarettes per day triples the risk! By adding other risk factors, you significantly multiply the negative effects on your heart health. Avoid even second hand smoke as it; too, can have a detrimental effect on a woman's heart.

When I had a private practice as a clinical hypnotherapist, I helped people who wanted to quit smoking find success. Integrity is a big issue for me, therefore; at that time, I was a non-smoker myself. Besides being a bad habit, people smoke for a variety of reasons; to celebrate, to relax, to de-stress, or when sad, depressed, and angry. If a client came to me and wanted to quit because their spouse or partner wanted them to stop, then I told the client the therapy wouldn't work. A person needs to be self-motivated. An example of a self-motivated reason to quit smoking is a desire for better health. See Appendix A for a "quit smoking" script that may help you to stop smoking, too.

Risk Factor—Obesity and Women

Obesity is a significant risk factor in heart disease for men. However, according to an eight-year study, women who are even mildly overweight dramatically increase their risk of heart attack when compared to men. Based on current statistics, 38 million women are overweight. In fact, the numbers on obesity are staggering. Obesity is a global problem, and by 2015, the WHO estimates that 2.3 billion will be overweight; of that number, 700 million are predicted to become obese (Lloyd-Jones et al., 2010).

I know that a woman's weight is a delicate subject — particularly when the media taunts us with wisp-thin women whose size we might only dream about — but we must reduce our girth, ladies. I enjoy good food and consider myself a connoisseur in the kitchen, but there are several issues that affect my eating, and thus my weight.

First, there are many women who like to eat at night, me included. What I realized is that during the long, Norwegian, summer days — where it can be daylight past 10:00 PM — I didn't eat as much, and I made healthier choices. However, during the winter months where the darkness lasted as long as the earlier summer sunlight, my eating changed significantly. During this time, I tend to have night cravings for high sugar-based food, which is unhealthy because sugar increases triglycerides and as a result, puts fat on the heart.

Another problem I had was staying up too late at night. Staying up late, or becoming sleep deprived, creates stress in the body, and it increases the secretions of cortisol, which comes from the adrenal glands. The increase in stress also may increase the desire to eat sugary snacks. Since I realized that I have a tendency toward seasonal affective disorder (SAD), I use a special "bright" light box that mimics outdoor light and may affect brain chemistry to decrease depression during darker seasons and gray days. I use mine regularly during the long Norwegian winter, and it has improved my mood and curbed my appetite, significantly.

The next step, of course, is to go to bed at a reasonable hour. People who already are stressed, which as we have seen both increases appetite and cortisol output, may find it difficult to do at first, but good habits can be developed. It's best to go to bed without a television on, in a comfortable bed, and in a darkened room. Sufficient sleep can do wonders to rest the mind as well as the body. Sleep also can help to decrease weight gain because it increases a hormone called leptin, which aids in weight loss.

The next thing to understand is that our stomachs are only as big as our fist. You are probably wondering how I know this tidbit of information, and it comes from attending several autopsies, while I was an EMT-D. As you eat your stomach will expand to approximately the size of your open hand. Wow! In comparison, think about the size of your fist; now picture what you would normally eat on a dinner plate. As you can see you are probably overeating when you compare your fist to the amount of food on your dinner plate. The key is to reduce your portion size and eat often.

Heart patients (and those who don't want to become heart patients) must eat small meals because the physical stress of a large meal is not good for the heart. **Use a salad or desert plate — rather than the generous sized dinner plate** — to promote healthier, smaller portions. My husband's answer to that advice is to pile the food higher on the small plate and go back for thirds. That's cheating, as I like to share with my patients' families.

Many cardiac patients tell me how hard it is to lose weight. I make weekly calls to those who are reducing because they need a support system. I coach their spouses, too. We all go together to the grocery to learn different ways of shopping for food.

Did you know that the best food for us is placed along the walls of the stores? There we'll find the most important food groups and the freshest foods. The center aisles have the most dangerous food because it's processed and contains additives that the human body just wasn't made to digest and use day after day. The body doesn't recognize it as food! If the product is in a package, box, bottle, or can, it most likely isn't healthy — especially when compared to fresh foods.

Every time we eat, we stimulate one of two hormones called glucagon and insulin. Glucagon is the fat burning hormone and insulin is the fat storage hormone. We want to stimulate glucagon, obviously. We can do this by eating a balanced diet of protein, complex carbohydrates, and appropriate sources of fat. On the other hand, to stimulate insulin, a good dosage of donuts, coffee with lots of sugar, a cola drink, and a desert of cake or pastry will do the trick! Too much insulin leads to diabetes for some people — for too many, in fact, as we'll talk about later in this section.

There are some great dietary programs to consider. Here are two that many cardiologists recommend:

❤ Nathan Pritikin's Program has been discussed and verified in over 100 studies in prestigious medical journals documenting its success. Pritikin was living proof that people can reverse heart disease through diet because he did that for himself. In fact, when he died, his autopsy revealed that his arteries were like a teenager's. *The Pritikin Edge: 10 Essential Ingredients for a Long and Delicious Life by Dr.* Robert A. Vogel is an excellent book.

❤ Dr. Dean Ornish also has written helpful, science-based books that might be useful: Dr. Dean Ornish's Program for Reversing Heart Disease: The Only System Scientifically Proven to Reverse Heart Disease Without Drugs or Surgery and Eat More, Weigh Less: Dr. Dean Ornish's Life Choice Program for Losing Weight Safely While Eating Abundantly.

Sodium intake and water retention go together. A high salt diet leads to water retention and all the discomfort and poor health that come with it — not to mention the unattractive effects on our bodies. One of my favorite cookbooks is *The Low Salt, Lowest Sodium Cookbook* by Donald Gazzaniga. It's a worthwhile book for reducing the salt and not cutting out the taste. Learn to cook with less or no salt. It's surprising that once I became used to a low salt diet, everything else tastes too salty and even unappetizing.

Of course, getting to the root of the problem of why we overeat is another issue — maybe the biggest. As a clinical hypnotherapist, I also had many weight-loss clients. The interesting thing about this work was that most of my clients had a psychological event tied to the eating behavior. That event triggered the food-consuming response, which led to the overweight. Once that psychological event was addressed, the eating behavior was no longer a problem.

While clinical hypnotherapy is one way to begin to heal in terms of an overweight body, we need to remember that it takes self-discipline, strong will, and a support system to be successful. As we reduce that girth, we need to master our minds. In doing so, we take control of our appetites and of our heart health.

See Appendix B for a "weight loss" script that can help you with the intellectual and emotional parts of losing weight.

Risk Factor—High Cholesterol Level in Women

Another well-known risk factor for heart attack is high cholesterol. Since women tend to have higher levels of HDL than men, the majority of heart health studies show this risk factor to be less evident in women as compared to men.

HDL is the high density lipoprotein, and it's the "good stuff." LDL is the low density lipoprotein, or the "bad stuff." To remember which is which when you look at your own lab reports (and you should *always* get copies of lab tests for your records), think of the word *heavenly* for HDL and the word *lethal* for LDL. As I discussed earlier, estrogen plays a key role in HDL for women and its presence is why women previously were thought to be protected from heart attacks. Additionally, women tend to lay down plaque evenly along the artery, whereas men have clumps of plaque. This difference in men and women can lead to misinterpreting an angiography in women.

As I explained in Chapter One, my tests revealed that my cholesterol levels were in the normal range, but I was given the maximum therapeutic dose of Lipitor anyway. The treatment protocol didn't consider my biology as a woman or as a woman with normal cholesterol levels. This drug made me deathly ill. I told my husband that if I had to live like this, then life was no longer worth living. My husband was scared when he heard me say those words. I was like a zombie, the living dead. It muddled my thoughts, left me completely breathless, no energy whatsoever and feeling rundown.

If I wasn't sick before I began that medication, I certainly was sick on it. I was so desperate to feel good, I started to skip the medicine every other day to see how I would feel. Amazingly better! *Ah ha*, I thought, *it's the drug*. But why was I prescribed this drug and why did I need the maximum dosage when I obviously didn't have a cholesterol problem? I asked my cardiologist these questions, and he told me that this medicine is a cardioprotective drug. However, it didn't help prevent the next heart attack. Instead, I had one that was seven times worse than the first.

I returned to my primary care doctor and told her that I was taking myself off Lipitor because of the way it made me feel. She suggested that I should not go off the cardioprotective completely and asked me to try simvastatin, the generic version of the brand-name drug Zocor. She prescribed the maximum dose again. I stayed on it for a few months and then my forearms started hurting, a ripping, burning sensation, however, the pain was much worse at night, and I began to wake up feeling as if someone was shredding my thigh muscle with a knife.

I started to wonder why I had this kind of pain and realized it might be the generic statin (simvastatin). During a follow-up visit, I told my doctor about my muscle symptoms. She seemed surprised but tried to reassure me that I was okay and that my muscles were not wasting away or being damaged. After all, your heart is a muscle too! When she asked me to stay on the medication, I said that if I had to be on this drug, I wanted to be on the name brand version. With Zocor, I found that I had fewer problems, but I still needed to titrate down to the lowest dose before I could tolerate it. Let's talk about name-brand versus generic. A generic drug is supposed to be a replica, chemically structured, as the name brand. I do not believe this is entirely accurate. If this were true, then I should not have felt any difference between the two drugs, simvastatin (generic) and Zocor (name brand). I know from manufacturing that although it may be the exact same ingredients on the label, the processes itself could be different, and different grade materials could be used to cost cuts. I had a conversation about this issue with my cardiologist and he agrees to use the name-brand instead of generic.

I have several points to this story:

💛 A one-size-fits-all treatment plan doesn't exist. Women may not tolerate the same amount or type of medication as men. Even without this difference between the sexes, no two people are biologically the same, and drug types and dosages may need to be changed.

💛 Various brands or versions of a drug may work differently, which means that we might have to try more than one type before experiencing success.

💛 Doctors don't know what we're experiencing as a result of a drug until we tell them. If a doctor seems to dismiss the symptoms, respectfully insist on being heard. Get a new doctor, if necessary.

💛 If high cholesterol is a problem, decrease those LDLs and increase the HDLs.

Natural ways to increase HDL are to lose weight, quit smoking, and exercise more. Remember that with exercise, the key is not intensity but time spent overall. Walking longer and slowly is better than racing to get the exercise done quickly. This is a case where there's no award for hurrying the process.

Risk Factor—Diabetes in Women

Women have an increased risk of a second heart attack if they have diabetes connected with lower HDL levels. However, diabetic men are not exposed to the same risk of a second heart attack under similar diabetes conditions and HDL levels. In the U. S., there are currently over 15.7 million people with diabetes of which 8.1 million are women. Of those cases in women, over 90% have Type 2 diabetes, which used to be known as "adult onset" diabetes.

The sad fact is that Type 2 diabetes, typically caused by lifestyle choices in diet and exercise, is affecting women at an epidemic rate. Although diabetic men and women share the increased risk of heart disease, men have experienced a higher survival rate, better quality of life, less risk of blindness, and a longer life expectancy as compared to women in recent years (CDC, 2001).

In fact, according to the latest studies, women have an increased mortality rate from heart disease when it's associated with diabetes and depression (more on depression in Chapter Seven). In addition, smoking, poor diet, and a sedentary lifestyle is linked with both depression and diabetes. Researchers speculate that these lifestyle risk factors could affect the nervous system and adversely affect the heart (Pan et al., 2011).

Risk Factor—Stress in Women

In 1974, Friedman and Rosenman published the best seller *Type-A Behavior and Your Heart,* which was recommended by many cardiologists at that time. As a teenager, I remember my father reading it, and his self-assessment was that he was a Type A. This book motivated many studies and quickly *Type A* was part of our everyday language. In 1989, Rosch took this idea a step further and proposed that Type A is self-perpetuating behavior because the stress of this behavior induces adrenaline, which correspondingly keeps the person working harder and harder. This idea makes sense to me. For example, when I was an EMT in my younger years, we used to joke about how we were all "adrenaline junkies" that got high from excitement waiting on the rigs for the next call.

There is a motto that a man works from sun up to sunset, but a women's work is never done. Today's contemporary women have it all: career, marriage, and family, and stress, stress, stress! Until recently, most studies related to stress and heart attacks have been focused primarily on men. Dr. Michelle Albert, a cardiologist at Brigham and Women's Hospital, is the senior author of a groundbreaking research about women and stress. She said, "women make up half of the workforce in this country," so the impact of job stress on their health is "an important issue for employers as well as employees" (Slopen et al., 2011).

Her landmark study followed 17,000 healthy women, a median age of fifty-seven, for ten years. The study found that women working under strain in high-pressure jobs have an overall 40% higher risk of heart problems, including heart attacks, strokes, or clogged arteries needing bypass surgery or an artery-opening angioplasty procedure. These figures strongly suggest that women need to reduce their stress at work and find relaxation whenever they can. The risks are unacceptably high, and life is too short to ignore the effects of stress — regardless of the job and even of one's desire to work.

Stress is serious. We need doctors to understand that helping women is not just about the physiology of the heart but the whole package — that a woman simply is different from a man. Women with heart issues are complex. We literally hold our emotions in our hearts. We can die of a broken heart. We can have our hearts wounded by an emotional trauma, which may take years to recover. Not only does our blood flow through our hearts, but so do our emotions and connections to the world. We need more research into how stress and emotions affect women's heart disease.

Risk Factor—Depression in Women

There are many studies (Doering & Eastwood, 2011; Monteleone, 2010; Jiang & Xiong, 2010; Whang et al., 2009; Burg & Abrams, 2001) that link depression and heart disease more strongly in women than in men. Anxiety also is linked to women who have suffered heart attacks. Anxiety is a normal reaction to a stressor.

Women's worries and anxieties may show up in the body through physical symptoms like back pain, sleeplessness, or stomach discomfort. However, for people who have had a heart attack, anxiety can affect us by manifesting as chest pain and subsequent heart attacks, as well as in the kinds of body/mind/spirit depression described in this chapter.

Anxiety related to heart attacks can manifest in various ways:

- 💜 *Physical effects:* heart palpitations, tachycardia (rapid heartbeat), muscle weakness, tension, fatigue, nausea, chest pain, shortness of breath, stomachaches, or headaches

- 💜 *Cognitive effects:* fear of dying, especially when pain exists

- 💜 *Emotional effects:* feelings of dread, trouble concentrating, tension, irritability, restlessness, or feeling scared

- 💜 *Behavioral effects:* becoming withdrawn, changes in sleep patterns, and nervous habits

The symptoms related to anxiety are so numerous that it's easy to mistake heart attack symptoms for anxiety symptoms. Just to see how complicated it can be to align the symptoms with the right cause, let's look at what type of anxiety is associated with the chest.

Anxiety symptoms commonly associated with the chest area:

- 💜 Chest pain or discomfort

- 💜 Concern about the heart

- 💜 Feeling like you have to force yourself to breathe

- 💜 Finding it hard to breathe, feeling smothered, and/or shortness of breath

- 💜 Heart palpitations where the heart beats too hard or too fast

- ❤ Irregular heart rhythms, fluttering or "skipped" beats, a tickle in the chest that leads to coughing

- ❤ Pounding heart or heart feeling as if it's beating too hard

- ❤ Rib or rib cage tightness, pressure, or feeling of a tight band around the rib cage

Clearly, there are many similarities between these anxiety symptoms and those of a heart attack. As we discussed in Chapter Four, these similar symptoms help to explain why so often women's heart attacks are misdiagnosed as simply a case of anxiety.

Depression and anxiety are two separate disorders, and it's possible to have one without the other or to have both. In the Nurses' Health Study from 1992 to 2004, scientists followed 63,000 women. The twelve-year study concluded that depressed women were more than twice as likely to experience sudden cardiac death caused by an irregular heartbeat. Additionally, depressed women were 40% more likely to die from heart disease compared to women without depression, according to Whang et al. (2009). One connection might be a link of taking antidepressant medications called SSRIs and an increased risk of heart attacks, as some recent research suggests (Whang et al., 2009; Kraztz et al., 2009).

Of course, more research is needed to determine the underlying causes of heart attack and multiple risk factors, including depression. It seems important to examine whether women are prescribed SSRIs for perimenopausal symptoms instead of considering bioidentical hormones, which are hormones that are synthesized from plant chemicals and are identical in molecular structure to the hormones women's bodies create. Sometimes, these are called "natural" hormones. In my case, my gynecologist had never heard of bioidentical hormones, and this is the case for a number of women with whom I have spoken. It's to our advantage to advocate for serious and extended research in this area.

In recent news pertaining to SSRIs and women who have had heart attacks, a word of caution seems necessary. Taking anticoagulant treatments and SSRIs is associated with increased bleeding according to according to a study (Labos et al., 2011). Not only is depression an issue after a heart attack, but this evidence suggests that depression also is a risk factor. Chapter Seven addresses depression as an issue post-heart attack.

Risk Factor—Body Size and Coronary Disease

As odd as this may sound, shorter women statistically have a greater chance of having a heart attack than a woman taller than 5 feet 4 inches or 1.64 meters. One British study published in *The Lancet Oncology* found that women over 5 feet 9 inches tall had a lower risk of heart disease and that taller women had an increased risk for cancer. A recent meta-analysis confirmed the relationship between body size and CHD, concluding that shorter women have a 50% higher risk of CHD than tall women (Paajanen, 2010).

There are several theories regarding these statistics.

1. Shorter women have smaller arteries, and smaller arteries may clog more easily.
2. Smaller women sometimes carry extra weigh in the midriff, which can lead to or be a sign of heart disease.
3. Taller women have lower blood cholesterol (Rich-Edwards, 1995).

These may be reasons that some women complain of chest pain, but have angiographies showing that the heart and vessels are clear. Such test results lead towards one-in-five women getting a referral to a psychiatrist or gastroenterologist rather than a cardiologist. According to researchers at the National Heart, Lung, and Blood Institute, some women's vessels are too small to be seen easily on an angiography, yet these small blood vessels can be constricting, clogged, and causing chest pain. These smaller vessels are located on the lower branches of the arteries.

I think it's pathetic to wish for a stent—but I did. When I had the second heart attack, I wished that I needed a stent to open my arteries because it would mean that the doctors had found the problem and had a way to fix it. However, my arteries were clear, no blockages. It was my good fortune that I didn't need a stent, but I was envious of my roommate who got one. The desire for a definite diagnosis can be overwhelming!

Because this woman was quite tall and her arteries were proportionately larger, she had a wrist (radial) angiography rather than the groin (inguinal) like me. She was up and about the day after her stent placement—my source of envy. But she also was smoking and eating potato chips, which I knew wasn't good for her. I asked the clinical interventionist if we could try a radial angiography, too, but it didn't work and we headed back to the groin. Slim women with fine structure and veins that roll are typically not good candidates for the radial angiography.

Risk Factor—Response to Treatment

Women are 12% more likely to die of a major heart attack at a hospital and less likely to survive than a man upon arriving at the hospital. They are more likely to die when leaving a hospital than a man. African American women have an even higher mortality rate than white women in short-term survival (surviving to leave the hospital) and long term survival.

Approximately 1% fewer women survive balloon angioplasty compared to men. Coronary Artery Bypass Graft (CABG) is twice as dangerous for women. In one study, researchers found that body mass made a difference in survival for women undergoing a CABG; the same body mass for a man didn't similarly affect male survival. It seems likely that the difference in survival rates is linked to a man's naturally larger arteries.

Women may not receive cardiac enzyme testing automatically upon entering a hospital with a possible heart attack. However, the cardiac troponins, or TnT levels, are essential for diagnosing heart attack, as I explained in Chapters One and Two. Be sure to insist on these tests especially if you are presenting with indigestion, mild pain between the shoulder blades, fatigue, and/or shortness of breath. There is no time to wait because waiting too long can cause irreparable damage to your heart.

> *Because a woman's heart attack symptoms are so similar to those of anxiety, it's important to insist on a cardiac enzyme test to check troponin levels in addition to other cardiac biomarkers.*

Risk Factor—Describing the Symptoms

I have saved this risk factor for last because it could be the greatest risk factor for women having heart attacks. This risk regards how women describe their symptoms, and it comes from misunderstandings about their symptoms. Although some women have more amorphous symptoms than men, who usually present with shoulder and chest pains, my experience is that women tend to describe any of their symptoms in less concrete and less urgent terms. Indeed, women seem to have a common inability to communicate their symptoms in a way that doctors can easily recognize as significant to the patient. This communication style may lead to misdiagnosis and delay in treatment.

For this reason, it's possible that any doctor's or hospital's initial response to women heart patients may be a reflection of the ways women present their symptoms.

Men tend to describe their experience using words like crushing, gripping, squeezing, pressure, chest pain, and profuse sweating. Men commonly use metaphors such as, it feels as if I have been run over by truck or there is an elephant sitting on my chest.

Women, on the other hand, tend to use words like it sort of feels as if you have heartburn, a burning sensation in my chest, kind of feels like mild pressure, I feel anxious, I have been having trouble sleeping, I have been tired, I have been feeling exhausted, and very fatigued.

We can see how these words will get women a prescription for antacid or something for panic attacks! Women need to use stronger, more urgent words like *a burning that is radiating from my sternum down my arms*, or *extreme fatigue to the point I cannot walk or breathe* that will more clearly indicate something is seriously wrong.

Let's complicate the picture a bit. Using Figure 4.1, look at the close relationship among the early warning signs of a heart attack, depression, anxiety, and menopause. The bold, capitalized text illustrates the repeated symptoms. As shown below there are striking similarities between the early warning signs of a heart attack in relation to depression, anxiety, and menopause. This relationship illustrates the importance of the way we communicate and the descriptors we use to describe our symptoms.

Figure 4.1: Relationship of symptoms among heart attack, depression, anxiety, and menopause

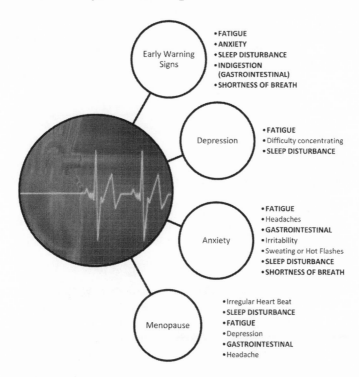

It's crucial to learn the best language for describing symptoms. A possible heart attack is not the time to be vague or too wish-washy.

My experience with female heart patients is that they tend to have a heightened awareness of their bodies, which could account for them seeking medical help quickly. Some women have symptoms a week prior to the onset of the initial heart attack. Such symptoms include:

- ❤ A sense of doom
- ❤ Trouble sleeping
- ❤ Fatigue
- ❤ Indigestion
- ❤ Anxiety

I also think women—in general—have a higher pain tolerance than men. For readers who have had a baby (or two or three), I think you might agree about this possibility. But, culturally speaking, women are taught not to complain and not to disagree with doctors. There's a common consensus that women should do as the doctor says. Even if we don't admit to this feeing, many of us wouldn't dare to question them or their diagnosis.

My own mother died because of this attitude, and I could tell stories of other women who suffered the wrong treatments because they were afraid to tell the doctor "no" or to ask for more time to talk about their needs. I have learned to look at this problem as one of self-advocacy. *The doctor works for me.* Caring for me is the doctor's job.

As part of this self-advocacy, though, we have to help our health care professionals to understand the exact symptoms. Just like an automobile mechanic can't run a diagnostic test on a car with a vague description of a problem, a doctor also can't figure out what tests to run without explicit descriptions of symptoms. If we don't use clear and descriptive words, the doctor may tell us to go home and return in a few weeks when the symptoms become more definitive. For cardiac arrest patients, that may be too late!

> ***Please remember:*** *If you don't present your symptoms in language that nurses and doctors recognize as typical of a heart attack, you may not receive the right tests and treatment. A medical professional determines whether you fit the cardiac protocols, so it's critical to communicate your symptoms clearly without downplaying them.*

Lessons Learned

1. Women are different from men in many different ways. Past studies of heart disease and drug development may not have recognized those differences. Ask your doctor how the diagnosis and prescribed treatments will affect your female body.

2. Women die from CHD at different rates than men. In fact, heart disease is the number one killer in women—much more so than breast cancer. At medical appointments, talk to your doctor about your risks for heart disease. Talk about:

    a) High blood pressure

    b) Smoking

    c) Weight

    d) Cholesterol levels (and understand your HDLs from your LDLs!)

    e) Diabetes

    f) Stress

    g) Depression

    h) Body size

    i) Response to treatment

3. Learn how to explain your symptoms—for any physical problem or unusual signs—in clear, detailed language. Communication is critical to having your illness correctly diagnosed in a timely way. One woman told me about her relative who went to the doctor complaining of vague

symptoms. She was referred to a psychiatrist and given an antidepressant. A week later, she died of a heart attack. Help yourself by using concrete words to describe your symptoms. See below.

Instead of saying this:	Say something like this:
It kind of feels like indigestion. (If you have a condition like gastro esophageal reflux disease [GERD], this sign of an MI may go undetected.)	I'm having symptoms of indigestion that are not normal for me.
I have a burning sensation in my chest.	My **(what)** chest is **(symptom)** burning mostly on my **(where)** left side.
It sort of feels like mild pressure.	I feel **(what)** pressure on my chest. OR It feels as if someone (or an elephant) is sitting on my chest.
I feel anxious	I have an overwhelming sense of impending doom.
I have been having trouble sleeping.	I have not slept well in weeks.
I have been tired OR I have been feeling exhausted OR there is fatigue.	I feel unusual fatigue, exhaustion, and/or shortness of breath that is not normal for me I am having difficulty breathing and complete exhaustion. From a scale of 1 to 10, ten being the worst. What is it?

4. Become a self-advocate. Women can be timid around doctors (even around female doctors), so:

    a) Prepare for the visit by taking a list of concerns and questions.

b) Take notes or bring along a family member or friend to record key messages from the visit.

c) Don't leave the visit until you are satisfied you have communicated your needs and understand the doctor's responses.

5. If you think you may have had a heart attack or symptoms of an impending heart attack, ask the doctor for a cardiac enzyme test to measure troponin levels. I can't stress enough that this test was the *only* way the doctors knew that I had suffered a heart attack given that my arteries were clear on both the angiographies.

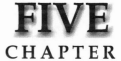

FIVE

CHAPTER

Research and Reflection

There are many ways to respond to the shock of a heart attack. One is to become internally focused and depressed. Another is to become angry and self-pitying. Yet another is to deny that anything has happened and to continue on with old habits and behaviors. Although I fell into the hole of depression and felt self-pity at times, I deliberately chose not to remain stuck in old behaviors. This chapter talks about some specific actions that we can take to help our bodies to heal.

Having an Advocate

After my second heart attack, I became acutely depressed. I felt as though I was living in a void, life was hollow and empty, like a bad dream. I was paralyzed with fear, anticipating the next attack that I perceived could happen at any time. Since I didn't know why I had heart problems to begin with, I had little confidence in the type of treatment I was receiving. Despite the fact, that I had the support of my family, I felt alone and disconnected from life. They could not understand the feelings of emptiness I described. For the first time, I actually understood what my father experienced mentally and emotionally. I needed help. There is no shame in asking for help. In fact, it is a strong person that recognizes they need help and asks for it.

Depression to the extent that I felt it is such a prominent problem for heart attack patients that I have devoted Chapter Seven to it. Given my professional background and personal makeup, one of the few actions I believed I could do was to research my condition. When we're feeling sick and emotionally depleted, researching may seem like too much work, so this is a chapter that should be shared with an advocate.

An advocate is anyone who can be our ears when we can't listen well, our eyes when looking at the small, or the big picture is extremely challenging, and our minds when our brains are too confused to interpret the world around us. I served as my father's advocate; for example, when he was exploring his options for coronary artery bypass graft and transplant surgeries. My husband and a close friend alternately were my advocates during the most difficult times of my heart condition. An advocate should accompany us to our appointments and consultations—especially in the hospital when receiving news of various tests. This person can ask questions that we've forgotten or not thought of and help clear up misunderstandings before they take hold and cause damage.

Just like we need them to help with our doctor's visits, we need our advocates to help with research into the illness. As patients, our mission is to get better. Sometimes we won't have the energy or focus to spend on research, but the more we know about our health problems and their possible treatments and prognosis, the more we can help ourselves to become better. Research is proactive.

Conducting Research

My own research began with trying to understand the tests and medication regimen that my doctors gave me.

For example, I needed to know more about the troponin tests and what its levels meant. These tests, remember are the only ones that initially showed positive results and revealed that I had, indeed, had heart attacks. During my research, I learned that the American College of Cardiology Committee considers cardiac troponins to be the preferred markers for detecting myocardial cell injury. The troponin I (cTnI) or T (cTnT) are the forms most frequently assessed. Typically, the troponin level rises from two-to-six hours after the initial injury (the heart attack itself), and it peaks within twelve-to-sixteen hours. The cTnI remains elevated for five-to-ten days, while the cTnT remains elevated for five-to-fourteen days.

The increase in my troponin levels were clear indicators of heart damage that could only have been caused by a heart attack. Given that the angiography didn't show heart damage, the troponin levels were crucial to doctors seeing my symptoms as part of real cardiac events and not as stress, anxiety, or hysteria.

Because these tests are so vital for diagnosis of cardiac injury, they are frequently updated and improved for sensitivity, so when we research, we need to look for the most current information. And, we may need to conduct research every few months to stay on top of new developments in heart disease science.

I also had a number of questions regarding the medication I was given. Since the doctors didn't know what caused my heart attacks, I sometimes felt as if medicine was being thrown at me without clear purpose just to see what stuck. I knew the doctors were following a standard treatment protocol and prescribing medicine with scientific reasoning, but I questioned how the standard treatment would be right when my heart wasn't showing typical or expected damage.

To be compliant, I began the medication regime as the doctors ordered. However, because we still didn't know *why* I was having these heart attacks, before I could know how to get better, I needed to understand why I was taking medication. Normally, I'm the one the family goes to for the medical research, but who was going to do it for me? I was tired and weak from the heart attacks and — it seemed — from the medication, and I found all the reading to be daunting. In fact, until my advocate started helping me, it was all the more depressing because I was doing the research for myself.

Reading

Reading all the statistics connected to heart disease is even more depressing. My father's experience with statistics regarding the lifespan of a heart transplant patient taught me that reading the statistics may not be beneficial when trying to recover. Since this information may even be somewhat suggestive, patients need to be careful about reading and digesting it when we are vulnerable. We need our advocates to help especially at this time. One thing that I became critically aware of is the degree of vulnerability to ones psyche after a heart attack. I was extremely careful not to be influenced while I was recovering.

But I'm headstrong, and I needed a mission to conquer my depression. It became my quest to find out what was wrong, and healing my heart became my primary focus and goal in life. I was obsessed — thinking and praying about healing morning, noon, and night. I was forced to act because of the threat of another attack. It seemed as though no one was doing anything for me — the doctors could only wait until the next heart attack to learn more about my case — so I had to do the work myself.

Since I knew I could not do it alone and be successful, I enlisted a close friend who is a proficient reader of scientific articles. She became my research partner, and together we did the research. Our goal was to prevent the next attack and heal my heart.

My friend's brilliant mind was critical because she could review the important from the unimportant in a plethora of medical information about heart attacks. She helped me to look both at traditional materials and at research focused on women. She also helped me to make decisions about which publications to read in terms of publication bias. Together we discussed whether the authors had a specific agenda (like pushing a particular surgical technique or preferring a medication brand or type) and she helped me to be wise about whether to accept the information as relevant to me.

Another thing my research partner did for me was to help me discern what was valuable to read since I was not strong enough to do it myself at the time. When reading about cardiac disease or any healthcare issue, it's always important to ask: *And how do you know this?* I like to go straight to the peer-reviewed journals as the original source. Under normal circumstances, I can decode the scientific language easily. Right after my heart attacks, though, my mind felt, muddy, foggy, and even simple articles were difficult to read. (That kind of cognitive fuzziness is common, by the way, and it usually goes away. If it doesn't, talk to your doctor about it.) In those cases, my research partner advocated for me by reading and explaining the research to me.

There's also a lot of information on the Internet, and not all of it is reliable. Be careful and discerning. It's too easy to get bogged down with everything we read, and a research partner can help us to exercise sound judgment. Since she lived in California, my partner read the data first and, through the magic of time zones and email, I had the necessary information to read by the time I woke up. Then we discussed it through email or telephone and decided whether it was worth looking into that subject more deeply.

One of the things I learned from the research was the value of good nutrition. To transform my body chemistry and bring myself back into balance, I decided to change my diet radically and to include only the healthy, fresh foods found along the walls of the grocery store and to include more fresh fish. My goal was to make healthy foods my "medicine cabinet." I decided to take nutritional supplements for the rest of the support my body needed. To do this, I sought the guidance of Dr. Steven Sinatra.

I read Dr. Sinatra's book The Sinatra Solution: Metabolic Cardiology and thought: Wow! This is the first cardiologist I've heard of who knows about supplements that are beneficial for the heart. I especially liked that he knew about the interactions between the drugs and the supplements. I was so impressed with Dr. Sinatra that I called his office to make an appointment. Although Dr. Sinatra was not taking any new patients, I sent in my information and told him all the medications I was taking. I explained my unusual case, and Dr. Sinatra took the time to recommend the nutritional supplements that I should be taking. By coincidence, these were exactly what I was taking. I felt relieved that I had gotten an expert opinion.

I tell this anecdote for three reasons.

1. We need to be careful combining natural supplements with heart medications. It's essential to get a knowledgeable health care provider's help with this goal.

2. It's helpful to get a second or even a third opinion from well-regarded doctors. Each time we tell
   our story to a new doctor, we can learn something
   different.

3. Don't be afraid to contact a famous doctor if you think
   she or he can help. If that person is too busy to see new
   patients, she or he will likely have the nursing staff share
   information or an opinion.

Charting

As soon as possible, I wanted to get off prescribed medications. I went to the health food store and bought hundreds
of dollars' worth of products. These would be expensive in
the U. S., but they are even more costly in Norway. I was
literally banking on nutritional supplements to help me get
better.

Kurt saw all the medications and supplements I was taking,
and he said: "How can you remember all the stuff you took the
day before? You should keep track of it and write it down." He
had a valid point. A chart would help me.

My mother had taught me her charting techniques many
years ago to help me find patterns of illness and behavior when
my children were small. I think she did it because she was somewhat forgetful, but keeping a chart leads to new ways of looking at symptoms and medications. This information can help to
understand one's illness from a different perspective and to solve
some puzzles.

I started to write down everything I ate and all medications
and supplements I was taking. I noted the time, amounts, and
observations about how I felt.

Example 5.1 shows one of my charts:

Monday, September 5, 2005			**PERIOD** **NITRO**
Observations: Indigestion, pain between shoulder blades while walking, sudden loss of energy, extreme fatigue. **TOOK** Nitro. Event lasted a few minutes. Day 2 of my period.			
Time	**Quantity**	**Description**	**Nitro/BP/Glucose, etc.**
0700	1	Soy Protein Shake w/Super Greens and a teaspoon of virgin coconut oil	109/70, pulse 73
	1	Chromium	
	150 mg	Q-10	
	2 grams	Vitamin C	
	400 mg	Magnesium	
	100 mg	OPC	
	MEDS	1-ASA 1-Cozaar + 1 Thyroid 75 mg Plavix 5 mg. Norvasc	
12:15	1	Fish salad	114/72, pulse 73
	1 gram	Vitamin C	
	1	Raw Carrot	
3:30	1	Salmon and Salad	
6:00	1	Greek Salad	
8:00	200mg	Magnesium	NITRO
	150 mg	Q-10	
	1 gram	Fish Oil	
	1	B-Vitamin	
	1	Folic Acid	
	1	Alpha Lipolic Acid	
	MEDS	5 mg Norvasc, etc	

This is an example of a simple chart, which includes observations, monitoring, and daily intake. You could also use a journal and divide the page into four sections:

1. Observations: Things you notice and feel, e.g., took nitro.
2. Monitoring: Your blood pressure, pulse, etc.
3. Daily Intake: Food list.
4. Meds and Supplements: List everything you take.

Be sure to indicate the days that nitro is needed. Use a red mark, or fold over a page corner, or a little note tab to find that notation easily when needed. Next, once a week, or every other week review your journal to look for patterns.

Example 5.2 presents a calendar chart. Use it to make a note of the days that nitro is needed for easy reference, for example. Then, return to the daily journal to determine whether there are patterns. Consistency in noting symptoms and medication is the key. For best results, document everything including how well you responded to the medication and how you felt afterwards.

Example 5.2

December 2011

Sun	Mon	Tue	Wed	Thurs	Fri	Sat
				1	2	3
4	5	6	7	8	9	10
11 Period START	12	13	14 NITRO	15	16 NITRO	17 Period END
18	19	20	21	22	23	24
25	26	27	28	29	30	31

In my charting strategy, I tried to use guidelines from a nursing approach called SOAP, which stands for Subjective, Objective, Assessment, and Plan. I altered the SOAP guidelines to do the charting myself. I changed the approach to a more personal one that required me to reflect on and evaluate my feelings and experiences, and to understand what I was doing about those things. Finally, it allowed me to summarize my observations about myself *and my body.*

Subjective: My experiences

1. Initial impressions of the medical situation
2. How I'm feeling
3. General observations and other noteworthy information regarding my sleeping, eating, symptoms, and so on

Objective: My self-assessment

1. My demographic information, especially age and gender
2. My major problem
3. My history of the present event
4. My previous medical history
5. My allergies

Assessment: Analyze my feelings and experiences

1. Rule out anything that may affect my treatment
2. Record how well I think I'm doing on treatment

Plan: Describe what I did

1. Record my actions chronologically
2. Describe the doctor's or my plan
3. Recap my current status
4. Record my action plan

This chart is beneficial not only for finding patterns, but also for helping us to learn to trust our emotions and physical experiences. With a chronic illness like heart disease, it can be remarkably easy to trust doctors more than ourselves. Yet, as patients, we need to remember that our doctors depend on us to provide them with accurate information about our experiences. Charts can help.

Appendix D provides a blank SOAP chart that you can copy and use. **Example 5.3: Example Completed SOAP Chart**

Subjective Feelings	Objective Experiences
In this section, I write down my chief experience or other things I was feeling.	*In this section, I do an objective self-assessment.*
Example: **Today, I was sad, because _____. This made me angry.**	*Example:* Today is **day 4 of my period**. *I'm having some* **chest pain**. 109/75, pulse 73
Assessment of the Feelings and Experiences	**Plan – Description of Actions**
In this section, I evaluate the significance of my recorded feelings and experiences.	In this section, I write down everything I did in chronological order.
Example:	**TIME 07:00** Soy Protein Shake w/Super Greens and a teaspoon of virgin coconut oil
I had chest pain today. To relieve it I took a squirt of **nitro** spray. After 5 minutes, the symptoms didn't go away, so I took another squirt and within 5 minutes, the pain was gone.	Chromium 150 mg Q-10 2 grams Vitamin C 400 mg Magnesium 100 mg OPC L-carnitine D-ribose
Next, I asked myself the following questions:	
What was I doing before I took the nitro?	**MEDS** 1-ASA 1-Cozaar + 1 Thyroid 75 mg Plavix 5 mg. Norvasc
What was I feeling emotionally today? Sad, anger, hurt, etc.?	**TIME 12:15**
Did I eat something that gave me indigestion?	Fish salad

If you are still menstruating, what day are you in your cycle?	1 gram Vitamin C 1 Raw Carrot
Overall Observations: *Example:*	**TIME 15:30** Salmon and Salad
*I had **chest pain**, took **nitro**, and was on my **period**.*	**TIME 6:00** Greek Salad
[In real life, these observations may have taken weeks or months to connect or understand.]	**TIME 8:00** 200mg Magnesium 150 mg Q-10 L-carnitine D-ribose 1 gram Fish Oil 1 B-Vitamin 1 Folic Acid 1 Alpha Lipolic Acid MEDS 5 mg Norvasc

It's easy to see that a chart provides tangible evidence in an objective and quantifiable form that doctors tend to believe. For example, charts can provide a stronger case if a medication change seems necessary.

Breakthrough

After months of charting, I noticed a pattern that seemed like a possible breakthrough. There was a pattern in the colored tabs I had placed on the edges of my journal pages. I placed a colored tab each time I started my menstrual period until the end of my cycle and a different colored tab when I used the nitro. I noticed that my heart attacks occurred in close relationship to my periods and that I took the nitro on the days I had my period. Next, I reflected back to the times I was in the hospital. I had my period the second time, and the first time I was in the hospital I had just finished it.

I theorized that my menstrual cycle and my heart attacks were connected. Given my age (a young 47years old at the time of the attacks); I knew that I was in the perimenopause phase (the beginning of menopause). We are taught that estrogen is a known cardioprotective in women and after 60 years old we have the same risk factor as a man for heart attacks. Therefore, I was perplexed why I was having attacks being so young; however, researchers believe that perimenopause leads to fluctuating hormonal levels and/or decreasing amounts of estrogen in a woman's body. During this phase, in my menstrual cycle and just prior to each heart attack, I felt as though I had cognitive problems — brain fog is how I would describe it. Normally, even during my periods, I had perfect memory and exceptional attention to detail. But prior to the heart attacks, I seemed forgetful, depressed, and generally not happy. I never had premenstrual syndrome (PMS) problems during this time other than low energy.

Part of my research process was to consult with numerous doctors and to present them with my charts and theories. When I sent my medical records, one prominent cardiologist from the U. S. said the following in an email dialogue:

Your arteries spasmed, and your type of heart attack (when all the tests are negative) accounts for .01% of all heart attacks. These types of heart attacks usually happen in women.

I wrote back and indicated that my heart attacks occurred around the time of my menstrual periods. He replied: *"Exactly, yes, when they [women] are stressed."* This cardiologist also recommended calcium channel blockers as a medication (not for high blood pressure in this case but for spasm). I was extremely excited to have some validation that I was on the right track with my search for patterns.

When I told my doctors about this hypothesis, one asked me: "Do you think you are that unique?" Stunned, I replied that all people are unique and that not everyone is going to have the same reasons for heart problems. There was complete silence. Then I told him that, in fact, a well-known cardiologist confirmed my hypothesis when he indicated the physical stress of my period is most likely connected to my heart attacks. He replied, "Well, then, I guess you have your answer."

Next, I spoke to my other cardiologist at the hospital; he was open to thinking out of the box and took an interest in my charting. In fact, when I showed him the pages, he reached over and took my journal to examine. I could see that he had a genuine interest in my research. He indicated that the supplements I was taking could be helpful and appreciated that I was researching non-medicinal options. I explained that my research suggested that the drugs he prescribed to me were not linked evidentially to positive effects on women. In fact, one of the studies clearly stated that more evidence was needed before prescribing one drug to women. Again, my words were met with silence. Then, he stated that these drugs were well-known cardioprotective medications. "Yes," I said, "for men."

Beyond talking to cardiologists, I needed to talk to my gynecologist since hormones and menstruation seemed to be a part of the equation. She replied that she had never read about a relationship among menstrual periods, hormonal fluctuation, and heart attacks in the medical journals. She talked with me about possible ways to avoid having a period as a protective against additional heart attacks. She recommended that I have an intrauterine device (IUD) inserted and implied that it would be a little painful, but since I had children, it wouldn't be a big deal. I declined that offer.

She didn't recommend hormone treatments, which was good because prescription hormone replacement therapy (HRT) is not advised by the American Heart Association. Yet I did want to balance my hormones if possible. One choice beyond HRT is Femarelle™, which is a selective estrogen receptor modulator and a super soy product. I am currently taking those two products right now, and it has been a lifesaver to get my hot flashes under control. Other supplements that I'm taking seem to be helping to balance my hormones.

However, I'm also interested in bioidentical hormones, which my gynecologist had never heard of either. For example, there is SottoPelle™ Therapy, which was founded by Gino Tutera, M.D., F.A.C.O.G. SottoPelle™, or biologically identical hormones, which are administered in what the researchers for this company consider the proper human ratio using absorbable subcutaneous (SC) pellets. By SC delivery, the body controls the release of hormones according to its need, which Tutera's company claims is closer to its natural action than any pill, patch, cream, or injection. Interestingly, this product is not just for women but for men, too. We must continue researching our options for hormone balancing as they become available in our local areas.

Decoding the Data and Where You Fit

It's essential to know yourself, your health patterns, and your specific type of angina.

There are five types of angina: unstable, stable, variant (or Prinzmetal), microvascular, and atypical. Having angina is not the same thing as having a heart attack. I think this is a little tricky because if this is your first time having any type of chest pain you are likely to think you are having a heart attack. I researched angina to figure out why I had the heart attacks, while having normal coronary tests. Let's review the information about angina and what it explains about my heart attacks.[5]

---

5 For more information, see http://www.nhlbi.nih.gov/health/health-topics/topics/angina/

1. **Stable:** Stable angina has a pattern or trigger and lasts for a short time. It can be induced by exercise, stress, extreme emotion, overexertion, overeating, and extreme cold or heat. It disappears when you rest or take medication for angina. Learning the pattern can help to minimize the symptoms of stable angina.
2. **Unstable:** Unstable angina has no pattern and is more serious. It should always be treated as a medical emergency. It may signal a heart attack and does not go away with rest or medication.
3. **Variant:** Also known as Prinzmetal angina, it usually occurs between midnight and early morning. It's very rare.
4. **Microvascular:** Also known as Syndrome X, it can be brought on by strenuous exercise.
5. **Atypical:** There is no pain and it produces so-called silent attacks, which may be due to higher pain thresholds. Atypical angina is more common in women. It may include a burning sensation, a sense of indigestion, extreme fatigue, and shortness of breath.

My first heart attack: The symptoms were vague. I knew that something was not right. My physical feeling was new to me, and it was unshakable. I knew I was not well. The sensations started with sharp, burning feeling, and then it became a knot the size of golf ball in the center of my chest. It wasn't truly painful; it was just there like indigestion, but I have never had indigestion like that and never in the morning on an empty stomach. I started sweating. Perhaps this could have been mistaken for a hot flash. I could see on Kurt's face that he was genuinely concerned that something was seriously wrong with me. He looked scared. I went upstairs to get ready to leave the house, and I was exhausted by the time I came down the stairs. For a split second, I thought about how strange it was to be so exhausted going down the stairs. By the time I got to the doctor's office, my symptoms were almost gone. The symptoms I had are considered atypical.

My second heart attack: The symptoms occurred suddenly while I was laughing and talking on the phone. It didn't go away with any rest, and any movement only made it worse. I knew there was no mistaking this feeling for indigestion; this was a full-blown heart attack. I had no nitroglycerine to take, so I took some baby aspirin. I think that all patients should be given nitro after the initial attack, as a protective measure for subsequent attacks. Additionally, these measures could potentially mitigate the damage caused by a heart attack. I believe this should be part of a standard protocol. The pain was strangulating my left arm, which felt as if I had on a tourniquet. There was tremendous pain and heaviness in my left arm and chest. When I reached medical help, I had two rounds of nitro and the pain was still there. This was clearly unstable angina.

Given the types of angina that I experienced and having a possible threat of another heart attack, I continued my research.

My third heart attack: During a leisure walk, a strange foreboding sensation came over me. I started burping. I had no pain. Suddenly, a wave of exhaustion came over me and stopped me in my tracks. I could see Kurt getting farther and farther away, and I could not keep up. He noticed I was lagging behind and walked a few paces back. We sat down by the side of the trail. I thought the fatigue would just leave, which was my denial of the event. I should have taken my nitro, but I didn't because I actually wasn't sure what was happening as it was even vaguer than the first attack. We were taught in EMT school that 50% of heart attacks are silent with no warnings or overt signs. Patients tend simply to collapse. Just as suddenly as the event began, it was over. It was the weekend, so I could not see my doctor then. I called in the next day and got a cTnT test, which confirmed that

I did have an episode although it was not severe enough to be in the hospital. I was relieved but worried for the next month. This third attack certainly was atypical.

Although learning about angina helped me to understand better how to classify my heart attacks, I was still somewhat puzzled as to why I had apparent normal coronary tests. Doctors suggested a number of theories but offered no certainty.

As I researched, I learned that women truly are different from men, even in the way they lay plaque along the arteries. In women, plaque may be distributed evenly along the coronary artery, which makes it undetectable in apparently normal angiography studies. Men, on the other hand, build up plaque like a bump in the road and the plaque is easily seen.

In women, plaque along the coronary arteries may not be visible in angiography studies unless a special ultrasound camera is used for intravascular imaging. The camera can see past the plaque and determine the actual wall of the artery. I wonder how many women leave the study thinking they are at low risk because their coronary arteries appeared to be perfectly normal. In fact, they are at *greater risk* because they are undiagnosed or not being treated at all.

The National Heart, Lung, and Blood Institute and the Women's Ischemia Syndrome Evaluation (WISE) studied ischemic heart disease and its pathophysiology in women. The WISE study goals were to investigate ways to enhance symptom assessment and cutting-edge diagnostic testing. Additionally, understand the origin of ischemia in the absence of coronary artery disease and to evaluate the impact of hormones in ischemic heart disease pathophysiology. The WISE study suggested that women who appear to have normal or clear coronary arteries may have *coronary microvascular syndrome*. When this syndrome is undiagnosed, the women who have it will continue to have symptoms, a declining quality of life, repeated hospitalizations, and more testing. Interestingly, the WISE study and St John Women Take Heart project agree that women have an increased risk when they show signs and symptoms of ischemia but without obstructive coronary artery disease (Gulati et al., 2009).

My charting, reading, and implementation of data to my case showed me that I was vulnerable for heart attacks around my menstrual cycle. The medical literature supported my theory and found that there was indeed a connection. The timing of the attacks and the pattern that it revealed was most intriguing to me. According to a Quebec study presented at the American Heart Association's Scientific Sessions (2000), women are more vulnerable to sudden, serious heart disease during the time of the menstrual cycle when their estrogen levels are lowest.

Researchers theorize that fluctuations of a form of estrogen reported in female test subjects occurred during and immediately after their menstrual periods. Psychological stress also may be related to estrogen deficiency in young women with coronary artery disease, according to the Journal of American College of Cardiology. "Now we're seeing that even young, premenopausal women lose protection from coronary artery disease when ovarian function and hormonal balances are disrupted," Dr. Bairey Merz said.[6] This means that even younger women may be at risk for the kinds of heart attacks I experienced.

As of today, I have been heart-attack free since September, 2005 and symptom free. For me, there seemed to be a direct correlation between my menstrual periods and the angina. I have remained on my core group of over-the-counter and supplementation products, which I believe is the foundation for my body's healing.

---

6 Dr. Bairey Merz is the Chair of the WISE initiative, Director of the Women's Heart Center and Director of the Preventive and Rehabilitative Cardiac Center, Cedars-Sinai Medical Center, Los Angeles, California.

Lessons Learned

1. Get an advocate who can be with you at hospital discharge, doctor's appointments, and in the library. You may need several advocates — that's okay. The job of these people is to help clarify instructions, to remember significant points, and to read and understand the research when we can't do it on our own.

2. Read and research. I read a lot and talked to other people after my heart attacks. Don't be afraid to communicate with other doctors, noted experts in the field, and other heart attack patients.

3. Meticulously document everything.

   a) When you chart your experiences, you don't have to be fancy. I chose to do it on paper because I have lost many important documents on my computer. I always take my chart — in whatever format — to my doctors to show them my symptoms and how I have been handling them.

   b) Help yourself and your doctor by looking for patterns in your chart and in your body's symptoms.

4. In summary, take control of the heart disease so it doesn't control you.

SIX

CHAPTER

Physical Recovery

R esearch after a heart attack can teach us many things about the risk factors — like those covered in Chapter Four — and how to help ourselves become better. There may be aspects of our physical lives that are moderately-to-wildly out-of-balance, and we may not even know it! This chapter explains some of the physical concerns that I learned I needed to address, and that may help you, too, in improving your own physical health after a heart attack.

Sleep Deprivation

Humans need daily sleep to stay healthy. Sleep rejuvenates their immune, musculoskeletal and other bodily systems and functions. Insufficient sleep is one possible cause of cardiovascular disease, suggesting that heart patients need sound and restful sleep more than ever. While entire books and studies have been addressed to sleep, in this book, I'll focus on one particular concern: the need for a sleep study.

> *Heart attack survivors need to have a sleep study!*

Although I had been telling my doctors for a few years that I had trouble sleeping — possibly due to perimenopause symptoms or life-related depression — nothing was ever done until I had the heart attacks. Then, my doctors recommended a sleep study.

Many times, sleep studies are done in a hospital or clinic setting, which isn't the most advantageous to sound sleep or what the patient might think is an accurate measurement of her typical quality of sleep. The test is called a polysomnogram. However, my test used a type of sleep strip and a recording device developed by Siemens, and it was conducted in the comfort of my own home. The results were surprising. I didn't have the obstruction typical of most cases of sleep apnea, but I had as many as sixty-to-seventy episodes when I stopped breathing during the night! That is sleep apnea, a condition by which the individual stops breathing temporarily (from a few seconds to a few minutes) up to thirty times per hour.

This vital news changed my life because the heart simply cannot be deprived of oxygen and remain healthy. In fact, researchers have done imaging studies of both the heart and brain after a heart attack and have found brain damage (Edelson, 2005). This research alone should scare all of us right into the sleep center without delay. Of course, like any research studies, these studies need further scientific validation and should be read for possible researcher bias, but the results they reveal make sense. In a heart attack, the heart stops working, which in turn stops sending oxygenated blood to the brain and body. Sleep apnea also results in a temporary but regular stoppage of oxygen to the heart and brain. Such an oxygen deprivation needs to be addressed.

I believe that a sleep study should be standard protocol for all heart patients. Years ago, I told my father that he needed to talk to the doctor about his snoring and the way he stopped breathing in his sleep. He wouldn't do it. One day, I took matters into my own hands, while he was sleeping; I audio-taped him and then played the recording for his doctor. Dad was furious, but I didn't care. It was horrible to hear and watch as he literally stopped breathing; then he started choking, gagging, and gasping for air. In the 1970s, doctors knew less about the connection between sleep and heart health. Sleep studies were not the norm. I told my father's doctor that I didn't think this kind of sleep and breathing stoppage could be beneficial for his heart. Interestingly, when my father had his heart transplant, he was put into a drug induced coma. We were told that the reason for this was to promote healing, and I suspect that it was helpful because he was on oxygen the entire time.

I'm amazed that when I speak to heart patients about sleep quality and sleep apnea they are surprised. Many have never heard of these problems, making me wonder why their doctors haven't discussed this issue. Let's be clear. You need a sleep study if you:

- ❤ Have had a heart attack
- ❤ Are tired during the day
- ❤ Have trouble sleeping at night

- ❤ Take catnaps during the day

- ❤ Are obese

- ❤ Wake up choking and gasping for air

- ❤ If you have atrial fibrillation

Insist on it. You need to rule out sleep apnea to make sure your heart and brain are getting oxygen during your entire sleep cycle.

The primary "cure" to sleep apnea is to wear a continuous positive airway pressure (CPAP) device. This device has a mask or nasal pillow that delivers pressurized air designed to keep the airways open during sleep. Many people complain that they cannot sleep with the mask on. At first, it was strange for me, too. Having the sound and feel of air pumping is odd. I also did not like the feeling that I was bloated with air, but that was just for the first week or so. The rate on my machine was set too high, instead of giving up; I simply extended the first phase of the process so that I was deeply asleep by the time the machine kicked in. It took me about two weeks to get used to the machine. After a while, you may find that, like me, you cannot sleep without it. Snoring is impossible to do with a CPAP. This machine provides both the oxygen we need and the peace of mind. If you have been prescribed such a CPAP machine, use it. Healing depends on doing as much as possible for your physical health. I can say that it is certainly not attractive or sexy. It is definitely a turn off. My biggest fear was that my kids would come into my bedroom, while I was sleeping with my CPAP, take a picture, and put it out on Facebook!

High Blood Pressure

High blood pressure (hypertension) is a known risk factor for heart attacks, as I explained in Chapter Four. Hypertension is now becoming a global epidemic. In fact, researchers from the PURE (Prospective Urban Rural Epidemiology) study now estimate that 40% of the world population has hypertension. There are several reasons for high blood pressure that include genetics, lifestyle, and secondary factors. Sometimes, the cause is unknown (of an unknown "etiology"). However, there are several changes we can do to improve high blood pressure. Let's look closer at both genetics and lifestyle choices.

Genetics

A recent study by Wain et al. (2011) represents a milestone in identifying new genetic variations that influence blood pressure. Researchers had already discovered twelve other gene variations and combined with the recent discovery of sixteen more have identified twenty-eight total gene regions. The international collaborative research involved 351 scientists in 24 countries and more than 270,000 people of European descent to find the genes that affect hypertension and hypotension (low blood pressure).

Researchers Franceschini et al. (2009) found a relationship between behavioral and socioeconomic factors that can alter the genetic effects on blood pressure. For example, they found that our genes can be influenced by our lifestyle choices like smoking, physical activity, and drinking alcohol. The study compared smokers and non-smokers, finding a relationship between smoking and the gene that interacts with diastolic blood pressure. Although there is much more for researchers to discover about genetics and high blood pressure, it seems clear that our lifestyle choices can affect both blood pressure and the genes connected to blood pressure in negative ways. Positive lifestyle choices also can affect blood pressure, and we should make wise choices to that end.

Lifestyle Choices

Lifestyle choices are another reason that people develop hypertension. These choices include poor eating habits, being overweight, consuming too much sodium (to include too many carbonated sodas, diet or regular), and exercising insufficiently or doing the wrong kind of exercise for your body.

To address lifestyle-induced high blood pressure and to help improve genetically based hypertension, there are many things we can do. First, let's look at height and weight and the corresponding body mass index (BMI).

The BMI can assess whether you are underweight, normal weight, overweight, or obese. It's used to determine the body fat based on height and weight; however, it doesn't directly calculate the percentage of body fat. The BMI is not a precise measurement, especially for athletes like performance and body builders because they typically have more muscle; since muscle weighs more than fat, this method would overestimate the amount of body fat. In addition, the BMI would overestimate body fat in pregnant women. Conversely, it would underestimate the body fat the elderly, those who cannot walk, or those with wasting muscles. However, for the average person it's a good measurement that indicates whether one needs to shed some body fat.

Calculate your BMI

Calculate Your BMI

Pounds & Inches:	Kilos & Meters:
♥ Multiply your height in inches by itself (squaring the original number); then multiply that total by the weight; then multiply the total by 703. ♥ BMI = (Weight in Pounds / (Height in inches x Height in inches) x 703	♥ Multiply your height in meters by itself (squaring the original number); then, multiply that total by the weight in kilos. ♥ BMI = (Weight in Kilograms / (Height in Meters x Height in Meters)

BMI Status:

❤ Underweight: Below 18.5

❤ Normal: 18.5 – 24.9

❤ Overweight: 25.0 – 29.9

❤ Obese: 30.0 and above

Or, find out your BMI using the handy chart found in Appendix E.

1. Find your weight in pounds, kilos, or stones,

2. Find your height, feet and inches, or meters, and

3. Determine your BMI.

Use your BMI as one of various indicators of your general health and risk for heart attack. Which lifestyle choices might need to be changed to improve your BMI?

Sodium Recommendations

In their 2010 Dietary Guidelines, the American Heart Association recommended a two-phase step-down program to reduce sodium. The first phase is to consume less than 2,300 mg per day, which frankly is too high. There is no biological necessity for this type of sodium intake, especially if you are a heart patient. The second phase recommends lowering sodium levels to 1,500 mg.

I mentioned earlier, "shopping the walls" for groceries is best because center aisles are where you will find all the processed foods. These foods account for 77% of the sodium consumed, according to the 2010 Dietary Guidelines. To meet 2010 Dietary Guidelines, the food industry and manufacturers will need to reformulate some of their foods by reducing sodium and finding sodium alternatives that will satisfy the consumers. While the American Heart Association's goal is that Americans will have reduced their sodium consumption to 1,500 mg by 2020. Please don't wait for 2020, start now!

Growing up we never had salt and pepper on the table. We grew up as avid label readers, but when we moved to Norway, content labels, except for ingredients were non-existent. Therefore, there was no way you can effectively calculate the sodium. In this example look at the ingredient list; if salt, sodium, monosodium glutamate (MSG), sodium citrate, sodium alginate, sodium hydroxide, and sodium phosphate are in the top ingredients, put it back! You need to take the time and start reading food labels more carefully. There is hidden sodium in almost everything that comes in a package, box, bottle, or can. You need to go back to basics and stop everything that has to do with convenience foods. For example, next time you go to the store, pick up a can of soup and look at the label. Below, is a typical soup can label.

Nutrition Facts*
Amount Per Serving (serving size) = 1 cup (240 ml)

Calories 90
Fat Calories 30
Total Fat 3g
Sat. Fat 1g
Cholesterol 25mg
Sodium 650mg
Total Carb. 10g
Sugars 3g
Protein 6g

Notice the small portion size; it is only one cup, which is considered a single serving. If you eat one cup as the suggested serving, then your sodium intake is 650 mg. However, if you eat two cups, the sodium intake is a whooping 1,300 mg.

I learned to flavor my food by using something spicy in place of salt. For example, instead of loading my baked potato with salted butter, salt, sour cream, and chives, I sprinkle a little cayenne or a favorite pepper with chives and a small dollop of sour cream. It's quite delicious, and I now prefer this over the butter and salt. There are several easy ways to reduce your sodium.

Numerous studies show that the Dietary Approaches to Stop Hypertension Diet, known as DASH diet, has been proven to reduce blood pressure within 14 days, even without lowering sodium intake. DASH was originally intended to lower blood pressure; however, the program also addresses weight loss. This diet is physician-recommended and sponsored by the National Institutes of Health.

This diet is rich in potassium, calcium, and magnesium — three things that are necessary to healthy blood pressure. In addition, it recommends high fiber, low-to-moderate fat, low-fat or nondairy foods, and plenty of fruits and vegetables.

Personally, I'm a follower of Donald A. Gazzaniga's *The No-Salt, Lowest-Sodium Cookbook*. Gazzaniga was a heart patient, too. He collapsed while rowing due to congestive heart failure. His doctors told him to watch his diet, and that he did. He learned that just taking the salt shaker off the table and out of the kitchen was not good enough (although it certainly was a start). As a heart patient, he was particularly interested in cooking and was highly motivated. He creates incredible recipes that are 70% lower in sodium (as low as 500 mg of sodium per day) than found in some of the contemporary low sodium cookbooks. As a result of Gazzaniga's remarkable diet, medication, and daily walks, he was taken off the transplant list.

Quite a few cardiac patients have told me about their success using Gazzaniga's low-sodium diet plan. I know one patient who attributes his success entirely to this cookbook. His initial ejection fraction (how much blood ejects from the left ventricle) was down to 10%, and he was extremely sick. A normal ejection fraction (EF) is 55%-70%.[7] However, he not only survived; but, he also increased his ejection fraction substantially and attributes his success solely to this diet.

Exercise

Over time, exercise can help to lower blood pressure naturally — both by conditioning the body, which also helps with weight loss. I have a pedometer that I use to count steps daily. My goal is 10,000 steps per day. I have done this walking exercise since my first heart attack. Strengthening our cardiovascular health is more beneficial than constantly obsessing about losing weight and starving ourselves. Focus on your heart and your weight loss will follow.

After a heart attack, it's essential to ask the doctor for advice about the kinds of exercise you are allowed to do. I like the idea

---

7 In medical reports, these numbers might be written as "LVEF=35%" for an EF of 35%.

of cardiac rehabilitation or cardiac rehab, because many people are afraid to start any kind of exercise – and they stay sedentary just when they need to be using their bodies to get better. Patients can be monitored and taught safe exercises and limitations with cardiac rehab.

Before starting any exercise program, check with your doctor. I have a tendency to go overboard and to overdo everything – it's that Type A personality of mine. Exercise is no exception. So, I constantly have to check myself that I'm not doing too much and that I'm exercising in the right order for me. For example, I always do aerobic exercise and keep my heart rate in a target area. At first, I noticed that my pulse was rather high, but I kept myself in my target zone. I knew what my normal target heart rate was before the heart attack but not after, which made me unsure of how much exercise I could or should actually do. Again, this is another reason to start cardiac rehab, to find out your target heart rate and know your limitations under supervision. A target heart rate is a zone of exertion where cardiovascular exercise is optimal. Wearing an exercise heart monitor can help you to attain and remain in that zone.

For example, the American Heart Association recommends 50% -75% of your maximum heart rate. Your maximum heart rate and mine will likely be different. It's crucial to stay in the zone that is right for you. Here is a way to calculate your own target heart rate.

1.   First, find the maximum heart rate for your age. The "220 standard" is 220 minus your age to equal your maximum heart rate.

   a) For a 54-year old person, the maximum heart rate would be 220-54=166. The maximum heart rate for someone who is 54 is 166.

2.   Next, calculate the maximum heart rate while exercising.

a) To calculate the low range, multiply the maximum heart rate x 0.50. Work it out: 166 x .50 = 83.

b) To calculate the high range, multiply the maximum heart rate x 0.75. Work it out: 166x .75 = 124.5.

3. This means that, for an optimal workout, your heart rate needs to be between 83 -124 beats per minute, which is your target heart zone while exercising if you are 54 years old.

Your doctor or cardiac rehab specialists can help you to find your target heart rate if you would like help.

Check with your doctor about your exercise routine!

As a general rule for me, if I can talk while I'm walking, running, or cycling I am not overexerting myself. You should not be huffing and puffing. Take the exercise slowly and build up to your target rate. You will find that over time your resting pulse will improve with exercise. After a few weeks of exercise, my pulse was becoming lower both at rest and during activity, and I was able to increase the intensity of my workout.

Breathing

Simple deep breathing can help to lower blood pressure naturally. Infants breathe deeply from their bellies, but adults learned long ago to breathe more shallowly from their chests. Deep belly-breathing is excellent for the body overall. Products like RESPeR-ATE™ have come onto the market to help those with high blood pressure or hypertension by using specific breathing techniques. Although somewhat costly, the electronic, computerized device can teach people to breathe more deeply and slowly, and it has been clinically tested for lowering blood pressure naturally.

I know several people who have tried this device and have been pleased with how well it has worked for them. When looking for RESPeRATE™ and other such devices, look for the U. S. Food and Drug Administration (FDA) approval.

Beyond such products, tai chi and yoga classes are excellent for opening the airways. Although both types of exercise include spirituality and meditation while stretching—all of which is beneficial for us—it's their focus on breathing that seems most important here. A good teacher can help you to breathe more deeply and healthfully. The bonus is that you can insert your own spiritual practices (or none) into the process.

Supplementation

Supplementing our diets with vitamins, minerals, antioxidants, and enzymes are becoming fairly common. This section describes a few of the supplements that may be helpful to some cardiac patients.

Remember, however, to take supplements only under the supervision of a knowledgeable heath care provider. Be aware that certain adverse reactions could occur when combining over-the-counter supplements with your heart medications. Additionally, certain food should not be eaten with heart medications. For example, grapefruit should not be consumed if you take any type of statin to lower your cholesterol, (i.e. Lipitor or Zocor), certain high blood pressure medications, (i.e. Cozaar plus), or certain calcium channel blockers, (i.e. Norvasc). There are more drugs and over the counter medications that interact with grapefruit. If you are on any heart medications, make sure you read the interaction section on the medication inserts.

It's possible that your cardiologist or internist may not be aware of the perceived benefits of various supplements. To that end, find a health care provider who understands your cardiac medications and complementary medicine. Doing so is part of creating a health care team that works specifically for your personal health goals. Finally, please check with your doctor and pharmacist before taking any supplement, to determine any contraindications (reasons not to take it) with your prescribed medications or with other supplements.

Antioxidants

Any of us who have been around for the past twenty years certainly have heard of antioxidants. There is little scientific doubt that antioxidants stop oxidation, which is a, natural chemical, process that can produce free radicals (oxidative stress), which starts a chain of events that lead to cell damage or death.

The easiest way to understand oxidation is to think of how an apple begins to turn brown when you slice it in half. The process by which the white flesh of the apple becomes brown is called oxidation. This oxidation can be counteracted with lemon, which can be considered an antioxidant.

Oxidative stress has been linked to heart disease, cancer, aging, and various chronic and degenerative diseases like Alzheimer's and Parkinson's. Even simple aging of the skin has been researched and considered a possible victim of oxidation and free radicals, which is why many skin products tout their anti aging properties from antioxidants. Free radical damage also can occur from contact with tobacco in smoking and second-hand smoke, as well as from other environmental factors like smog, chemicals, and radiation.

To prevent such damage and to promote better health, some scientists suggest the supplemental use of antioxidants. For example, glutathione often is regarded as the mother of all antioxidants and is composed of amino acids glutamic acid, cysteine, and glycine. Glutathione is considered to protect cells from cellular damage, disease, and aging. Glutathione levels become depleted from oxidation, free radicals, stress, chemicals, illness, and the aging process.

However, how the body ingests the glutathione matters a great deal. Researchers Witschi et al. (1992) indicated that a single dose of three grams of glutathione, taken orally, failed to increase circulating glutathione to a clinically beneficial level. This finding indicates that oral supplementation is not effective in raising glutathione levels. Also, your level of SAM-e (S-adenosyl methionine) has a direct correlation to your glutathione levels. Instead, to obtain sufficient glutathione, you need to eat right and/or supplement it by prescription, IV, transdermal patches or SAM-e, which converts to glutathione. Again, do your research.

One scientific belief about antioxidants is that the amount of antioxidants we have in our bodies is directly proportional to how long we will live and our quality of life. On the other hand, some scientists believe that the stasis of antioxidants is more important than an overabundance. Like many complex medical issues, there are opposing beliefs. Therefore, I strongly recommend reading some of the studies with a reliable research partner and making decisions about taking antioxidant supplements in coordination with your health care providers. I prefer to eat my antioxidants instead of taking pills.

Although the body has mechanisms in place to squelch free radial damage, unfortunately, it's not enough. A good way to augment your antioxidants supply naturally is through your diet. Haytowitz and Bhagwat (2010) provide a comprehensive description of foods and their antioxidant capacities. There is mounting evidence to support the relationship between free radical damage and cardiovascular tissue injury in the human body. In the brain, evidence suggests that increased free radicals may be associated with age-related diminished brain functions and other disorders such as Parkinson's and Alzheimer's. Therefore, decreasing free radicals through our food simply makes sense.

Currently, the USDA recommends a daily intake of 3000-5000 ORAC value of antioxidants. ORAC means Oxygen Radical Absorbance Capacity; it is a chemical assay used to measure antioxidant values.[8] The higher the ORAC score means that it increases its potential to destroy free radicals. Foods that are high in ORAC are high in antioxidants. Studies suggest that eating fruits and vegetable with high ORAC values may help to decelerate the aging process in both the brain and body, according to the Jean Mayer USDA Human Nutrition Research Center on Aging at Tufts University (Prior et al., 1999). In fact, some researchers believe that certain combinations of foods have more cellular protection than the same foods eaten alone (Cao et al., 1995).

Below are a few examples of fruits and vegetables and their total ORAC values taken from the 2010 USDA Database for the Oxygen Radical Absorbance Capacity (ORAC) of Selected Foods.[9]

Fruit	Total ORAC μmol TE/100 g
Acai fruit pulp/skin, powder	102700
Apples, Red Delicious, raw. with skin	4275
Blackberries, raw	5905
Blueberries, wild, raw	9621
Chokeberry, raw	16062
Cranberries, raw	9090

---

8 ORAC was developed by Guohua Cao, a visiting scientist at the National Institute on Aging in Baltimore, Maryland.

9 Source: USDA Database for the Oxygen Radical Absorbance Capacity (ORAC) of Selected Foods, Release 2 - Prepared by Nutrient Data Laboratory, Beltsville Human Nutrition Research Center (BHNRC), Agricultural Research Service (ARS), U.S. Department of Agriculture (USDA) - May 2010

Currants, European black raw	7957
Elderberries, raw	14697
Juice, black raspberry	10460
Oranges, raw, all commercial varieties	2103
Pears, green cultivars, with peel, raw	2201
Plums, raw	6100
Raisins, seedless	3406
Raspberries, raw	5065
Strawberries, raw	4302
Tangerines, (mandarin oranges), raw	1627

Vegetables	Total ORAC μmol TE/100 g
Artichokes, Ocean Mist, boiled	9416
Beans, lima, immature seeds, canned, regular pack, solids and liquids	243
Broccoli, boiled	2160
Broccoli, raw	1510
Cabbage, red, boiled	3145
Cabbage, red, raw	2496
Carrots, boiled	326
Carrots, raw	697
Corn, sweet, yellow, raw	728

Garlic, raw	5708
Leeks	569
Lettuce, butterhead (includes boston and bibb types), raw	1423
Lettuce, red leaf, raw	2426
Onions, yellow, sauteed	1220
Peppers, sweet, green, raw	935
Potatoes, red, flesh and skin, baked	1326
Potatoes, Russet, flesh and skin, baked	1680
Spinach, frozen, chopped or leaf, unprepared	1687
Sweet potato, baked in skin	2115
Sweet potato, cooked, boiled, without skin	766
Tomato products, canned, sauce	694

Dark Chocolate

There are numerous studies about the good benefits of healthy dark chocolate, especially for women. However, not all dark chocolate is created equally and may be packed with calories, fat and sugar. Chocolate losses some of its antioxidant capacity through a process called *dutching*, which is used to reduce the acidity. Unlike traditional companies that use the *dutching* process, there is another company that uses a cold-pressed process to ensure that the beneficial antioxidant properties are intact. This company takes it a step further and tests its chocolate to receive an ORAC score. I cannot say what others have experienced eating this chocolate, but I can tell you my experience. I developed plantar fasciitis, which means an inflammation of the plantar fascia on the bottom of the foot. It was very painful to walk and stand. I went to specialists, and doctors, had expensive custom soles made, did all the exercises and even had cortisone shots. Nothing worked to reduce the pain. I had it for over a year until I started eating the healthy chocolate. I started eating 3 pieces a day, within a week; the reduction in my pain intensity was significantly reduced. Thinking more is better, I increased to twice the amount, in less than two weeks, and I was pain free. Once I was pain free I reduced the amount that kept me pain free. This product intrigued me, I investigated the company, met the owners, read all the peer reviewed journals that I could find. I can only say good and positive things about this company, the management, and the products. If you are going to eat chocolate, do your research and find the healthiest chocolate product for you.

Coenzyme Q10

Coenzyme Q10 (CoQ10 or Q10) is a catalyst that creates energy on a cellular level and is essential to produce ATP (adenosine triphosphate). ATP is like our battery of life and is produced in the mitochondria of cells. CoQ10 is needed for mitochondrial ATP synthesis. Ubiquinone and ubiquinol are both forms of CoQ10, but ubiquinone is the form of CoQ10 that commonly is found in stores. Ubiquinone is in the oxidative form and, when taken, it's converted into the reduced form of CoQ10 called ubiquinol. CoQ10 also works as an antioxidant.

In the late 1950s, Dr. F. Crane discovered an orange substance on beef heart mitochondria. Dr. Karl Folkers, a distinguished biomedical scientist, and his co-workers at Merck & Co. identified the structure and synthesized CoQ10 from it.

Their research led to the discovery that CoQ10 strengthens the heart muscle and energizes the cardiovascular system. Folkers believed that deficiencies in CoQ10 could be one cause of heart disease and that supplementation could help to prevent heart problems. Myocardial biopsies done on patients with various cardiac diseases have shown that there was a deficiency of the enzyme in 50-75% of the patients studied. As we age, our levels are significantly reduced, and oxidative stress can further reduce the supply of CoQ10.

Researchers in Japan have used CoQ10 as an approved therapy for heart failure since 1974 (Tran et al. 2001; Kettawan et al. 2007). The largest number of mitochondria and the greatest amount of CoQ10 resides in the heart and liver. CoQ10 is highly concentrated in the heart muscle because of its high energy demands and it's an essential nutrient. Folkers et al. (1990) warned that heart disease is caused by declining levels of CoQ10 and that it worsens with the use of statins. Recall that statins are used to correct high cholesterol and often are prescribed for heart attack patients.

Statin-induced depletion of CoQ10 is well supported by peer reviewed research. An FDA docket, exhibit A (2002) by cardiologist Peter H. Langsjoen, advised that a black box warning should be placed on all statins sold in the USA that reads:

Warning

HMG CoA reductase inhibitors block the endogenous biosynthesis of an essential cofactor, coenzyme Q10, required for energy production. A deficiency of coenzyme Q10 is associated with impairment of myocardial function, with liver dysfunction and with myopathies (including cardiomyopathy and congestive heart failure). All patients taking HMG CoA reductase inhibitors should therefore be advised to take 100 to 200 mg per day of supplemental coenzyme Q10. (Langsjoen, 2002).

As of the writing of this book, ten years have passed, and no black box warning about a deficiency of coenzyme Q10 has been placed on statins.[10] At the same time, the public doesn't generally know that CoQ10 is an essential nutrient for heart health. My point here is that readers need to talk to their doctors about supplementing with CoQ10, especially if they are on statin therapy.

There have been many patients who have told me that they take CoQ10 and many other nutritional supplements; however, some have said that they won't report it to their physicians for fear of being ostracized, belittled, or berated. We must be able to tell our doctors what we are taking so that we can get their advice. Unfortunately, many doctors are not educated in various nutritional supplements, yet I think the way of the future is to integrate complementary and allopathic (traditional) medicine. The patients of tomorrow will be active participants in their own health, as we should be now. If we are to create personal medical teams that can work with our specific needs, doctors must learn about these supplements and how they can interact with prescription drugs.

Magnesium

Magnesium is an essential mineral for the heart, muscles, and kidneys. One study showed that in post-menopausal women, a magnesium deficiency compromised cardiovascular health and glycemic (blood sugar) control (Nielsen et al., 2007). After my initial heart attack, my cardiologist advised me to take magnesium supplements because he believes that all women typically are deficient in magnesium. One interesting thing that I have noticed since I started taking magnesium is that I no longer have heart palpitations. In addition, 70% dark chocolate is high in magnesium, which is another good benefit for dark, not milk chocolate.

---

10 Interestingly, in February 2012, the U. S. Food and Drug Administration (FDA) added warnings about diabetes and memory loss to the packaging of statins.

Nattokinase or K2

Nattokinase (Natto) is an anti-clotting enzyme complex extracted and highly purified from a traditional Japanese food called Natto. Natto has been in the Japanese culture for more than 1,000 years. It's a type of fermented cheese-like food, which results in the creation of nattokinase enzyme based on the bacteria present on soybeans. It has been used as a remedy for heart and vascular diseases. Similar to serrapeptase, research also has shown that nattokinase aids the body in breaking down and dissolving the unhealthy coagulation of blood. Natto is a blood thinner. When I take Natto I do not use aspirin. A word of caution in taking any supplement, you need to check with your doctor or pharmacist about the potential interactions with your nutritional supplements and cardiac medications, especially if you have been prescribed Plavix (clopidogrel bisulfate), Coumadin (warfarin), aspirin (acetylsalicylic acid or ASA) or any of these combinations. If you have any unexplained bruising, for example, behind the knees, the stomach area, bleeding gums or unusual bruising not caused by an injury, you need to see your doctor, and please be honest about what you are taking! I had bruising all over, behind my knees in the crease, both arms and stomach area. I could barely brush my teeth because my gums were bleeding so badly. I knew this was not normal! I showed my cardiologist, and the look of shock on his face said it all. He immediate took me off Plavix and aspirin. I knew I needed some type of anti-clotting and this is when I discovered Natto.

Many patients have told me that they are taking, fish oil, Plavix, aspirin and natto. Some take Coumadin in combination with the natural products and wonder why their PT/INR (prothrombin time (PT) test is out of the target range. Just because something is potentially good for your heart does not mean you should take it. Be careful and do your research.

An older gentleman went to the emergency room complaining of chest pain. He thought he was having a heart attack. However, he was hemorrhaging internally and severely anemic because he combined his prescription drugs with other natural anti-clotting properties. Again, please talk to your doctor or pharmacist about this combination. If you are taking natural anti-clotting supplement you should still insist on getting a PT/INR test just make sure you are in the safe range. Patients do not like to tell their doctors because they feel belittled, and foolish by the way some doctors react. Communication is essential!

Books to Aid in Healing the Body from Heart Attack

Although there are many, many books to choose from in the heart health section of your local or online book store, I have found a few that have helped me most significantly. If your favorite book isn't listed here, that doesn't mean there's anything wrong with it; it only means that there wasn't enough room to address all the potentially helpful resources in this book. Please feel free to email your favorite book titles to me, at my website: www.dorinaerbo.com, so I can learn from its wisdom and perhaps share the book with others.

The Sinatra Solution: Metabolic Cardiology

In *The Sinatra Solution*, Cardiologist Dr. Stephen T. Sinatra discussed the importance of energy metabolism on cardiovascular health and the positive impact these three energy-supplying nutrients have on the cardiovascular system. He guides the reader through the basics of energy metabolism and cardiac bioenergetics, and clearly explained the role of coenzyme Q10, L-carnitine, and D-ribose in the body and specifically how they affect heart health.

The Hormone Solution: Stay Younger Longer with Natural Hormone and Nutrition Therapies

Several patients—primarily male doctors seeking stem cell treatments—brought *The Hormone Solution* to my attention. They were interested in this book because of the heart's hormone receptors. One doctor told me that he was reading Dr. Thierry Hertoghe's book because of the testosterone receptors located in the heart. He wanted to make sure before he came for his cardiovascular stem cell therapy, he was fully optimized so that he could potentially get the maximum results. As we know, hormones play a protective role in our health; in men, its testosterone and in women, its estrogen. For women, Hertoghe discussed the importance of a natural form of progesterone to protect the arteries from spasms. As we already know, there are many women who have heart attacks without obstruction of the coronary artery, me included. This fascinating book is based on thirty-five years of scientific investigation into weight management, foods that heal, and the foods that correspond to the hormones.

Reverse Heart Disease Now: Stop Deadly Cardiovascular Plaque Before It's Too Late

Reverse Heart Disease Now is another helpful book by Drs. Stephen T. Sinatra and James C. Roberts, two leading cardiologists, who collectively have fifty years of clinical experience. The book focuses on how the arteries become clogged and how to get them unclogged through medication, supplements, and diet. What I like about this book is that these two cardiologists understand typical heart medications as well as the supplement types needed to support heart health.

The No-Salt, Lowest-Sodium Cookbook

The No-Salt, Lowest-Sodium Cookbook is recommended by more of my cardiac patients than any other book. Many of these patients were relatively nonresponsive to medical treatment and on maximum medications. Some were told they would not live beyond five years, yet ten and fifteen years later they are still alive. My curiosity was piqued, and I had to read the book! The author, Donald A. Gazzaniga suffered from congestive heart failure and was placed on a transplant list. He was told that he needed to manage his sodium while waiting to move up the list. As he waited, he found a way to create fantastic dishes and menus with as little as 500 mg of sodium. I have tried his recipes, and they are very tasty. This is an absolute must-have book.

Biology of Belief

The Biology of Belief is a particularly fascinating book. I found out about it while listening to a podcast. One thing that stuck me was that the author, Bruce H. Lipton, Ph.D., was a former medical school professor and research scientist. During the podcast, he spoke about his petri-dish experiments and how cells would change because of their environment. Lipton's professor and mentor explained to him that it was necessary to look at an ailing cells' environment—not the cell itself—for the cause of its problems. This idea struck me as perfectly sensible. To explain my response, I've often wondered why some autologous stem cell cardiac patients do extremely well while others don't. One thing I have noticed is that those who become healthier demonstrate a profound belief that if they get the cells they need, they will be healed. Although, some may say this is a placebo effect, I think not, after five years.

They possess a positive mental attitude with a burning desire to become healthy again. Those who emphatically believe in potential healing seem to have the most extraordinary physical changes. Lipton explained that the cells are affected by the signals outside them—by their environment—including positive and negative thoughts. If the cells are affected by the signals outside them, (internal environment) then it would be plausible that if we optimized the environment, through positive lifestyle changes, medication and / or supplements, the environment could be enhanced to peak performance. I attribute my success to optimization of my body, mind and spirit. I believe this combination is critical for optimal healing and long term success.

Lessons Learned

1. If you're still alive after a heart attack, consider the event a very loud wake-up call to change your lifestyle.

    a) If you smoke, STOP! Kicking the habit is one of the most beneficial things you can positively do to influence your heart health.

    b) If you're overweight, lose weight under your doctor's supervision. Eat right and give your heart the right nutrition. See the book list for more information.

    c) If you currently don't exercise, start to exercise under your doctor's supervision or cardiac rehab.

2. Have a sleep study done to determine whether you're getting enough oxygen when you sleep.

3. Reduce your sodium intake. Remember, where salt goes water follows. Fluid retention puts a strain on your heart, which is a valid reason to check your weight every day.

4. Research by looking into books, peer reviewed journals and other literature that can help in your quest for better health.

5. Keep a journal of your progress toward better health. This activity is both good therapy, and it can help in expressing emotions that occur after a heart attack.

PART TWO

THE MIND AND SPIRIT
JOURNEY

SEVEN

CHAPTER

Depression: More than the Blahs

Depression is such a big issue for women who have had heart attacks that this chapter is dedicated to some of its symptoms and ways to move beyond it. Depression often is characterized by feelings of sadness, despair, discouragement, and a sense of powerlessness to change anything in one's world. Some of its symptoms include fatigue, sleep disturbances, and eating difficulties. Depression can be either situational or clinical.

A situational depression often occurs with illness and grief. In fact, heart disease is an illness that can lead to grief because it represents a loss of health, among other things. Situational depressions often disappear by doing the hard, emotional work of confronting the reality of the issue that has caused it and embracing the depression as a way of learning how to move through the problem. This chapter will be most helpful to those of us who are experiencing such a situational depression with our heart disease.

A clinical depression often looks like the kind of situational depression that comes with illness and grief. However, pervasive, oppressive sadness and a personal history with clinical depression are clear signs that you need to see your doctor and talk about possible medical help. Clinical depression is physically brain-based as well as emotional. If you and your health care provider determine that medication is necessary, then it is essential to work together on your plan for the depression.

In the case of clinical depression, some of the suggestions in this chapter may help with changing behaviors and thinking, but it also requires teamwork with your doctor or other health care professionals.

Depression Takes Hold

The connection among heart disease, depression, anxiety, and menopause makes this subject of depression more complex and even more crucial to talk about with relation to the body/mind/spirit connection—the primary theme of this section of the book. The body deals out the heart attack, but the mind and spirit can *both* contribute to illness *and* help the body to heal.

As I said in Chapter Five, a heart attack can bring on a sense of depression that is difficult to shake.

I wanted to think that my first heart attack was a fluke, an isolated incident never to happen again. I considered myself to be extraordinarily lucky that I had a sensitive awareness of my body and that my previous training as an EMT-D had kicked in when I felt those first symptoms. The self-awareness and training helped me to see my symptoms as acute, which got me access to the hospital quickly. So, I congratulated myself on my knowledge and actions.

But I also used this heart attack as a wakeup call to change some behaviors. Afterwards, I was a "good girl," followed the doctor's orders, and took all my medications. I ate fish almost every day—easy to do in Norway—took a few supplements, and joined a gym to workout. Everything seemed to be going well.

Six weeks later, I had the second and third heart attacks. I felt betrayed when I learned that the second one was seven times stronger than the first. I was confused, distraught, angry, and grieving that my hearth health was deteriorating, and no one knew why.

When I came home from the hospital the second time, it was a letdown. While I was glad to be out of the hospital, it felt foreign to be home. I felt sorry for myself and wondered "*why me?*" Tears of fear and pain eventually turned into tears of pity. I was on a downward spiral of despair and frustration. I was scared to be alone because I was afraid that I would have another heart attack, and no one would know. I wish I could turn my mind off and think about something else, but fear crept into my head and prevailed like a black cloud. My body's weakness and my mind's fears were entwined.

Soon, I learned how my spirit had connected with my mind and body in dealing with my heart disease. One night, shortly after the second heart attack, I had a dream that my dead brother Donny came to visit me. In the dream, I asked him what was wrong with me. He made a face of disgust and said: "Ugh. Don't stand too close to me. The stress is pouring off of you."

I said, "How do I fix it?"

He replied, "You have to fix yourself and get back into balance." Then, he left and wouldn't let me follow him.

I woke up immediately and thought the dream was strange. Donny's message wasn't too odd, though. There are many ways to interpret dreams, and we don't need to go into them here. But for me, my dreams are how my spirit speaks through my subconscious mind. In this case, Donny told me what I already knew deep inside: I needed to get myself back together again. I needed to release some of the stress, in my dream, that Donny found so repellant about being around me, and I needed to find balance in my life.

Finding balance was easier said than done and I became even more deeply depressed.

The Body/Mind/Spirit Connection to Depression

What does it mean to have a body, mind, and spirit connection to depression? In this case, remember that we're talking specifically about a situational depression that follows or precedes having a heart attack. The heart attack is physical. Sometimes a connected depression can have physical origins, too.

The Body

Before my heart attacks, I started noticing subtle changes in my body that signaled perimenopause. During this phase of life, a woman's hormones fluctuate and increase her chances of depression. Over a few years, I had gone to my doctor several times and complained about sleep problems; I just was not getting proper rest. The sleep disturbances took a toll after time, and it led to me telling my primary doctor that I was depressed. The doctor's response was that I didn't look depressed.

My doctor wasn't right, but he wasn't being insensitive. Heart disease can be a somewhat hidden illness in that when the heart is doing well, the patient also looks well — blood is pumping adequately, and the body is refreshed and oxygenated with each heartbeat. With depression, too, there are times when a person can look bright and alert, yet can feel dull, unfocused, and unhappy. We can use our minds to affect how we look and to control the emotions that we let the world see. I knew that a doctor couldn't diagnose depression just by looking at me even though what I looked like was an important indicator. Like many people, I wore a perkier face when I was out and about.

On my doctor's advice, after my heart attacks, I tried taking an antidepressant medication. There are times when our brains might be chemically imbalanced and clinically or chronically depressed; this is a physical or "body" issue. In these cases, depression often can be aided by selective serotonin reuptake inhibitors, or SSRIs (commonly prescribed antidepressants). When prescribed appropriately and used properly, these medications can relieve some depression and help us to feel more like ourselves again.

I reviewed the side effects of the prescribed medication and, quite frankly, was reluctant to try the SSRI. I used it for a few weeks and then stopped taking it. I'm aware that it can take up to six or more weeks before an antidepressant's best effects can manifest in the body. Given how many medications I was on and my personal dislike of taking medications to begin with, I simply didn't want to continue the treatment that long. Especially when my other cardiologist found out, he said, did you see the side effects? His eyes got wide, and his disapproving brow said it all.

Please note that I made this decision based on my belief that my depression was situational — a combination of the heart disease and grief over the changes in my life. My personal health history and the onset of the depression around the time of these heart attacks convinced me that I was not experiencing a clinical, body-based depression. **However, please do not use my personal decision as the basis for your choice about depression and medications. Please make your decisions about antidepressants by talking with your doctor(s).** Together you can make the right decisions for your situation.

I decided to tackle my depression from the standpoint of my mind and my spirit.

The Mind

The way a person interprets information is to some degree inherited or learned. The left brain deals with logic and the right brain deals with emotions. The so-called "primitive brain" is responsible for all the autonomic functions, such as heart beats and breathing. It's this part of the brain that keeps us safe, interprets danger, and takes control in fight-or-flight situations. The primitive brain is the autopilot of the mind's command center. We also have what is sometimes called a "higher brain" that decodes, analyzes, and assimilates information.

The mind responds to stimuli and has many ways to express itself. For example, we can go on a roller coaster for the first time and be extremely scared; this is the primitive brain reacting. The reaction can cause physical distress like inability to breathe and nausea. Over time, it's possible to desensitize ourselves to a roller coaster ride. Then, the higher brain is in charge, telling the primitive brain that we really are okay, and the ride actually is fun. Physical reactions change with the mind's change.

What happens to your mind when the news of a heart attack is delivered? When someone suffers a heart attack or any type of trauma, a sense of devastation can follow. The body sends out signals, and the mind must react to process what just happened.

If you've had a heart attack, think back to your first reaction. Mine was shock, disbelief, confusion, fear, and a distorted sense of having a bad dream that I couldn't quite shake off. I had to hear the news twice! I felt as if I had been given a death sentence. My primitive brain was at work. Was yours?

What happens next? We try to make sense of the news, understand the diagnosis, and start to cope. There is no script for being told you had a heart attack, and we must learn how to deal with the reality of an MI and the part of the heart that has died. We fear that life will change forever. We wonder about the severity of the heart attack, lifespan, and mortality. Grief begins. At the same time, we may be thankful to be alive, and the mind skips ahead looking at the heart attack optimistically as a wakeup call: *Of course, there are things I can do to change! I'll start right now.* The primitive brain begins grieving and the higher brain begins thinking logically, if somewhat shakily.

When we are forced to change, how do we respond? Most people behave in one of two ways—acceptance or defeat. Some people see the glass as half full and others as half empty. Which glass is yours? Maybe right now you feel defeat, but you probably want to move forward and don't know how. Realize that your body may not ever be 100% fully recovered. You may have to slow down a bit, change jobs or tasks on the job, revamp lifestyle, and do some healthy things that you have never thought about before. But as a heart attack survivor, you still have the opportunity to do them. How you look at and deal with all these changes, will impact your health. Your higher brain is working on these problems.

Our minds begin a coping process that was induced by the stress of the heart attack. The Elisabeth Kűbler-Ross model of how some people grieve describes five possible phases of grief *that can occur in any order and at any time after bad news*:

Denial: People may express a sense that what is happening is inconceivable. Or, they may say they're fine, when it's clear that they're not fine at all.

Anger: People may wonder *"why me?"* and blame others, especially God. Anger often signals a feeling that this heart attack is just not fair.

Bargaining: People may suddenly understand the importance of time and try to negotiate for a better deal, thinking *"Please let me live long enough to see my grandchildren."*

Depression: People may fall into the quagmire of depression, feeling like life is not worth living and any attempt is wasted. They may withdraw, cry, and stop communicating with others.

Acceptance: People may come to recognize that life is as it should be and that they'll be okay. They may decide that they will survive and begin to act positively to improve their health situation.

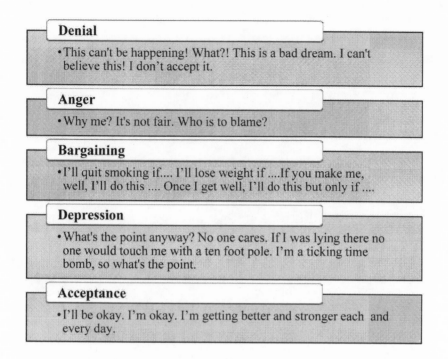

Denial
- This can't be happening! What?! This is a bad dream. I can't believe this! I don't accept it.

Anger
- Why me? It's not fair. Who is to blame?

Bargaining
- I'll quit smoking if.... I'll lose weight if ....If you make me, well, I'll do this .... Once I get well, I'll do this but only if ....

Depression
- What's the point anyway? No one cares. If I was lying there no one would touch me with a ten foot pole. I'm a ticking time bomb, so what's the point.

Acceptance
- I'll be okay. I'm okay. I'm getting better and stronger each and every day.

Figure 7.1: Some Phases of Grief (based on Kübler-Ross model)

Once we begin to accept what has happened—whenever that occurs—our expressions can be a combination of *thinking* and *physical action*, which engages the higher brain. For example, after I had the heart attacks, my initial reaction was one of anguish, but soon I began to take the necessary steps to correct what had happened. In fact, once our minds have made conscious choices, we typically follow those decisions with physical actions that put them into play.

Clearly, our minds can be "made up," which means that the mind has made a *choice*. Our minds also can *feel*. Emotional responses are common in depression following a heart attack. We "feel" sad, sorry, frustrated, afraid, angry, troubled, attacked, and wounded, for example. Let's keep these two functions of the mind—*choosing* and *feeling*—separate for a few minutes.

After I tried and dismissed the antidepressant medicine—believing that my depression was situational in nature—I decided that I had two choices. I could sit around and feel sorry for myself, or I could get up, start researching, and figure out why I had the heart attacks. This goal became my diversion to keep my mind occupied and to leave me no time to dwell on depression. I decided I could learn what I could do to heal myself. As I explained in Chapter Five, I *felt* depressed—those feelings couldn't be simply turned on and off. In response, I *chose* to be an active participant in my healthcare, which was a series of actions. I kept myself busy, and the research I did took my mind off my fears, self-pity, and general sadness. I used that negative energy—which *is* energy after all—and turned it into something positive. I looked for the proverbial silver lining in the dark cloud.

Remember that if you are clinically depressed, you cannot simply "decide" not to be depressed. In that case, you may not be able to take action in the ways this chapter describes. See your doctor to discuss whether your post-heart attack depression is clinical or situational.

The Spirit

People perceive of their spiritual selves in different ways, of course. Sadly, some people deny that they have a spirit because they're afraid of linking themselves to any sort of religious belief system. When I talk about the spirit here, I'm not suggesting that people have to have a particular belief system. The spiritual realm has to do with belief and faith in ourselves and—I think—in someone or something bigger than us.

What seems relevant here is to recognize that, as humans, we are physical beings (body) with minds that think (choice) and feel (emotions), and that we possess a spiritual nature (belief and faith) that looks both inside and outside itself for completion and a sense of wholeness. Often, that sense of wholeness is what is missing in our wellness.

Women often hold their worlds in their hearts. All their feelings and emotions reside in the emotional center of the body — the heart. Sadness, loss, and grief caused by instances like death, familial disconnect, divorce, job loss, and the like often are described by women as *heartache*. But more than feelings reside in the heart. The spirit often is described as residing there, too. What is a "hole in the heart" other than a sense of some essential element of one's personal world being missing? That component often is understood to be *love*. For many, love is the essence of the spirit. Without it, we feel less than human.

When we are depressed for any reason, it's sometimes linked to a sense of not being loved or not being loveable. Many people express that they feel less loveable when they are sick, as if the illness is a punishment from someone we love. And that is a problem of the spirit, which can be addressed by the belief and faith that comes with a healthy spiritual life. When your spirit is empty or incomplete, it's difficult to feel well in the mind and body. The connections among body/mind/spirit, therefore, are clear. The problem of depression can affect us in all of these areas after the devastation of a heart attack.

The Depression/Anxiety/Menopause Connection

In Figure 7.2, notice the relationship and the similarities among depression, anxiety, and menopause. The circle in the middle depicts the shared symptoms among these physical and mental experiences. In cases where a woman is experiencing two or three of these conditions at once, the result can be compounded symptoms where she may feel unable to change what she's experiencing physically or mentally. These shared symptoms of depression, anxiety, and menopause are experienced more intensely. Altogether, they can create a situation where a woman can become very ill and not know why she's suddenly so vulnerable to physical discomfort and emotional outbursts. These conditions not only can mask heart disease, but they can — as shown in Chapter Four — be risk factors for a woman's heart attack.

Figure 7.2: Connections among Depression, Anxiety, and Menopause

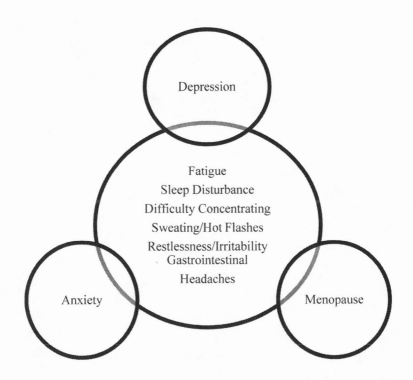

Taking Control of Depression

Depression can occur after losing a job, divorce, moving to a new area, the death of a loved one, and upon the onset of an illness.

You may have feelings of sadness, hopelessness, and you may feel unmotivated, and disinterested in life in general. If you are depressed or anxious, please don't be afraid to seek help from a professional. Asking for help is taking self-initiative, which can be difficult when we're depressed, but it's extremely beneficial for women who are heart patients to get professional help with depression. Learn whether your sadness represents situational or clinical depression. Find out whether medication, therapy, support groups, and/or other assistance will be suitable for you. You have a choice in how you deal with the depression although sometimes it's hard to see clearly.

> ***Please don't be afraid to reach out for help.***

I remember one day when I was so filled with emotion, I ended up on the doorstep of an American woman I know in Varhaug. I thought I was going there just for a visit and to have a cup of coffee. But when she opened the door, suddenly I became overwhelmed with emotion and started sobbing in her doorway. Embarrassed, I apologized for the emotional outbreak, and she reached out her arms and gave me an enormous hug. We talked for a long time, and I shared my story over coffee. Remarkably, I felt better. This improvement mostly happened because she was there for me and able to listen. It is a huge burden to carry so much emotion after a heart attack. My friend reached out to me and helped me to feel understood and not so alone. That visit was enough to give me the courage to move forward in my journey of heart health.

Remember that I believed my depression was more situational than clinical. I saw my getting better as part of a series of choices I was making about my health. Once I decided that I was no longer going to be depressed about my heart attacks, I began to take control of my emotions by sharing them more with others. Over the weeks, and months that went by, I got stronger, and I started to feel more like my old self again. I was starting to become happy again. It took some work every day.

Please remember, though, that if you are clinically depressed, you and your doctor will need to work together with your depression. There's no shame in having either kind of depression.

This next section is directed towards women with situational depression although some of the activities might help any depressed person.

Thinking Positive

Positive thinking is a mindset. We have a choice in almost every situation we encounter. But thinking positively can be hard. It takes determination and strong will. Positive thinking can help to address both the emotions and the physical symptoms of depression following a heart attack.

How many times do you wish for something only to be disappointed? Wishing doesn't manifest anything without action. It's essential to see yourself already healed and to feel — literally feel — that sense of wellness. You need to bring up the emotion that is connected with what a healed heart would feel like. Then, you can transform your healing by using your emotions and thinking. Here's how this technique worked for me. I practiced visualization to connect with my mind and spirit. In meditative states, I saw my heart as completely healed. I wasn't *wishing* for it to happen. I was *seeing* my heart as *already healed*. My vision was an expectation of healing, and I believe it helped lead to the real healing I later experienced.

Here is another example of positive thinking. When I felt low or fearful, I practiced diversion techniques. My favorite diversion was an appreciation activity. As negative feelings emerged, I would stop whatever I was doing and look outside in nature to appreciate. Living by the water as I do, I looked to the ocean or to a magnificent sailing ship or to the sun sparkling off the water. A tree with variegated leaf colors in the fall or the quiet hush of the night after a snowfall can capture my gratitude and hold it for some time.

Another way to redirect my negative emotions was to think of a time when I had been extremely happy, and then I held that thought for several minutes. Usually, this action cleared my mind and lifted up my emotions so I could think more clearly. For another example, every time I sensed my own fear, I replaced it with at least ten good thoughts. Not only did the good thoughts do a lot to deflect the negative feelings, but the cognitive act of counting those ten thoughts (and holding them in my mind) kept my mind busy enough to dismiss the negative feelings.

My favorite diversion technique is to use a rubber band around my wrist. If I think of something negative, I snap it—not too hard but hard enough to feel it. The brain doesn't like pain, so snapping the rubber band when a negative thought comes teaches the brain not to think negatively. The reward, of course, is the lack of pain when thinking positively. This method also works for smoking or any other thing one is trying not to think of such as those sugary or salty snacks that we're choosing not to eat anymore. At the time of my heart attack-related depression, I was still on blood thinners, so I couldn't snap myself because it would bruise me terribly. Please don't use this method if you are on any blood thinners!

Music is a powerful diversion. It is surprising when you listen to a song from your teen years, how those feelings and emotions well up inside you. I am instantly transported back in time when I play music that makes me feel young and vibrant. If you want to feel joy, use the power of music, but make sure you use the right music. As you know, music can trigger powerful emotions both positively and negatively. Choose music that uplifts you and brings you to place of happiness and feeling strong. One thing you can do is go for an enjoyable stroll listening to your favorite music that makes you feel alive and healthy.

Getting Support

Although these are excellent strategies for working with heart-related depression, we don't have to heal all on our own. It's often necessary to bring in a professional therapist or other people. Other ways to help ourselves after a heart attack include a support group for other survivors of heart attacks. Support groups allow people to talk about their experiences quite freely with others who understand because they, too, have experienced an MI or some similar heart disease. I believe that a useful support group is monitored by a trained facilitator who can ensure that everyone gets a chance to talk and that the group environment isn't a negative experience. The leader also needs to have a positive attitude about heart healing and should be someone who understands and knows what participants are experiencing on some level.

Making Positive Choices

Making positive choices and using such strategies may be difficult at first because we feel emotionally vulnerable after the heart attack, and any physical weakness contributes to this feeling. However, it is critical and of considerable importance to strengthen the psyche. Such strengthening becomes a habit of mind, and it can help to keep us healthy in the future and to heal faster in the event of future heart health problems.

Although this may be easier said than done, I believe that whatever your mind can believe your body will achieve. During the early 1990s while I was in graduate school for clinical psychology,

I had a private practice as a certified clinical hypnotherapist. From this experience, I created powerful self-healing scripting for myself. During my meditations, I used my scripts twice a day until it became engrained in my consciousness. Then it was easier to make the changes that needed to occur. Appendixes A and B provide two such scripts to stop smoking and lose weight—both of which are necessary lifestyle changes that heart patients need to make.

Beyond meditation, it's essential to find something that you love to do—something that makes you feel good. Think back to a time when something you did gave you pleasure, peace, or joy. What was it? For me, it was when I had a horse throughout my teenage years. Those were some of my happiest times. Riding my horse alone on country trails reconnected me with myself and nature. As a teen, I rode every day, feeling peace and joy. Now, I only have to smell horses, and it takes me back to that time and space.

After my heart attacks and when I was well enough to travel, my youngest daughter, and I went to Amsterdam, where we bought a Kossack Russian Arabian mare. She was a gorgeous bay mare in foal. In the mornings, I had a routine of cleaning stalls, feeding, and watering. After a few months, I realized just how therapeutic it was for me to take care of the horse. I actually found pleasure in mucking stalls because my mind was still and only treasured memories arose. Having a horse got me up, out of bed, out of the house, and back into nature. It was a grounding experience that returned me to a time and place when I was most at peace and happy.

Whatever it is that you liked to do in an earlier, perhaps happier time—maybe walking, creative writing, drawing, painting, or some other hobbies—try to find your way back to it. That activity can help you to reconnect with yourself and take you on the road to feeling well again.

Finding Self-Love

When people explore or work with their feelings after a significant emotional event like a heart attack, it often happens that old, unresolved pain emerges. In my case, I emotionally replayed some of the devastation of the double funeral of my beloved mother and younger brother, Donny. I re-experienced other hard times, too. After meditation one day, I realized that I still harbored deep anger about my job loss. These adverse experiences lurked deep in my spirit waiting to be healed.

Others have experienced such reconnection with heartbreak. For example, I spoke to a woman with familial heart disease. She had lost several family members — including her son — to cardiomyopathy. One of her greatest regrets was that she was not with her son when he died, having just stepped out of the room. We used clinical hypnotherapy, during a phone conversation, to return her to that time so that she could say goodbye. My point in telling this story is that if you are depressed about losing a loved one, home, job, or marriage, you still can get closure with professional help.

Do you remember what it felt like to fall in love for the first time? Do you remember how you felt when you were near this person? Every thought was consumed with this person's looks, smells, words, and mannerisms. You were utterly enamored. Women are full of feelings. Especially when depressed, we need to remember what is like to love again. Only this time, we need to be the focus of our own love.

A heart attack is a traumatic experience, but worse is a life without self-love. Love yourself like you never loved anyone before. Love is a powerful emotion that has the potential to heal, while self-hate, disgust, or even disinterest can lead to *disease* — which literally means *lack of ease* — in the body.

Lessons Learned

1. Depression is a powerful, negative experience that can manifest in the body, mind, and spirit. Often, it needs to be healed from all of these perspectives.

2. Heart attacks can lead to depression as the body is weakened and the mind and spirit must deal with this shock to their systems.

3. Depression, anxiety, and menopause have some similar symptoms — as previously described in Chapter Four — so it's necessary to keep a journal to track these symptoms for possible patterns. Periodically reflect and see whether there were certain triggers that may be responsible for those symptoms or patterns. Seek the help of your doctor, a psychologist, or another health care professional. It's essential to know your history, which will help your doctor to determine or rule out certain conditions.

4. Positive thinking is a mindset that we all can cultivate. It takes the desire to feel better and the discipline to act on it.

5. Sometimes we need professional help to move beyond depression. Such help may include a doctor's plan, antidepressant medication, support groups, psychological counseling, behavioral counseling, and/or clinical hypnotherapy.

6. In the end, self-love is critical to healing both depression and from a heart attack. While it's easy to feel wounded or angry at ourselves for having imperfect bodies, it's important to love the bodies we have and improve what we can through positive thinking and actions.

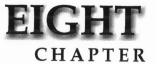

CHAPTER

Foundations for Healing

W hile doctors can do many things to help us to heal, the main power to heal is within ourselves. We are responsible for what we can do to encourage our own good health. As Chapter Seven revealed, the body/mind/spirit connection is critical to self-healing. This chapter explores foundational ways to engage the body/mind/spirit in healing after a heart attack.

The Napoleon Hill Roadmap to Health

Napoleon Hill was born in an impoverished family in 1883 and died a well-known personal development and financial advisor in 1970. The principles that he espoused as written with Andrew Carnegie as *The Law of Success* in 1928 were the foundations for self-help books and lectures. Hill's book *Think and Grow Rich* is a timeless classic and is still a top 10 best-seller, 70 years after publication. Napoleon Hill and W. Clement Stone co-authored the *Positive Mental Attitude, Science of Success*. Stone was instrumental in founding the Napoleon Hill Foundation, which is located at the world-renowned Purdue Calumet University and University of Virginia, College at Wise. I use Hill's principles for success in this chapter to convey some of the ways our thoughts can help us to become healthy again.

Although the language that Napoleon Hill used might seem somewhat old fashioned, his ideas are still as helpful today as they were when he developed them. Most of us will recognize the premises from contemporary approaches to the body/mind/spirit. In this sense, Hill is very modern, and these concepts can be applied to healing after heart attack. While men certainly can benefit from the strategies for healing that Hill's principles suggest, they are especially suited to the woman who is healing from a heart attack. I hope that they inspire you as much as they have inspired me.

According to Hill, to be healthy and happy, it's necessary to have a positive mental attitude, the first of his seventeen principles.[11] This positive mental attitude is aided most by having a "goal purpose," the "maintenance of sound health," a "mastermind group" (or some kind of help and support), and "applied faith spirit." The need for a goal, good health, group support, and applied faith is necessary in achieving a positive mental attitude.

Figure 8.1 shows these concepts as they relate to a positive mental attitude.

---

11 See Appendix E for all of Napoleon Hill's seventeen principles.

Figure 8.1: Components of a Positive Mental Attitude

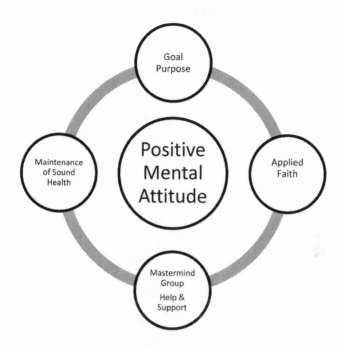

Positive Mental Attitude

Hill once said, "A positive mind looks for ways it can be done; a negative mind looks for all the ways it can't be done."

Nobody wants a heart attack. Even if our health and lifestyle habits haven't been optimal, we never planned to have a heart attack. Most people certainly want to get better. However, there are two types of patients: one that commits and one that does not commit. For example, they will both say they want to be healthy and well again, however, one patient does everything humanly possible to make it happen; while the other patient doesn't put in the effort.

Perhaps you're thinking: *"Hey, wait a minute. I didn't ask for any of this! Of course, I want to get better."* Yes, we all want to recover, but are we enabling it to happen? Are our actions and beliefs characteristic of a positive mental attitude that encourages healing? We enact whatever we subconsciously believe. So, if we don't *believe we can heal,* healing most likely won't occur. Similarly, if we don't want to make the lifestyle changes that enable healing, most likely, we will not get well.

Think of your health as dependent on a scale where you can have a positive or a negative mental attitude. Figure 8.2 shows a scale that is tipped just slightly toward a positive mental attitude (PMA). It includes wisdom, applied faith, sound mental and physical health, and peace of mind. Whereas, a negative mental attitude (NMA), on the other hand, is comprised of worry, fear, and misery. The Napoleon Hill roadmap to health requires that we tip the health scale toward a positive mental attitude.

Figure 8.2: Health Positive Mental Attitude and Negative Mental Attitude

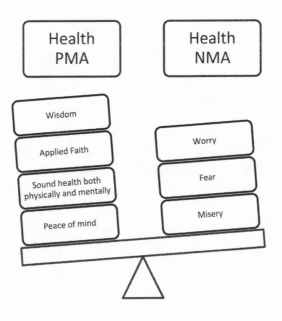

It's crucial to shift the scale's balance towards having a health-conscious, positive mental attitude. If you don't attempt to do this, you will develop and/or reinforce a negative health consciousness. Such a negative outlook naturally is strengthened by negative habits of thought, which then become the dominate thought pattern. Just as there are equal and opposing forces—right/wrong, good/evil, up/down, day/ night, positive/negative—there are a positive and negative health consciousness.

To develop a positive mental attitude, it's important to become aware of your thought patterns. Then, as soon as you think of something negative, replace it with something positive. For example, here is a negative statement: *I'm worried about having another heart attack.* State this idea more positively: *I'm doing everything in my power to prevent another heart attack.* Do you see the difference? The next move, of course, is to take the necessary steps to develop sound mental and physical health.

One way to create this mental shift regarding health is by discerning your primary purpose, a support structure, and applied faith. Together, these can lead to sound health, as I describe below.

Major Purpose

What is your primary goal regarding your heart health? In this book, I have assumed that the purpose is to achieve sound health by recovering from the heart attack(s) and setting up a healthier future.

My goal after the heart attacks was to heal myself to whatever degree was possible. I knew that doctors could only do so much for me, but I was at peace with that knowledge because I also believed that I could use my own body/mind/spirit connection to heal myself. I became passionate about my self-healing, getting better, becoming healthy and whole again, became my only thought and my primary focus.

Having a major purpose is the starting point towards achieving anything, according to Hill. He encouraged people to begin with one focused goal. Although many people will say, "don't put all your eggs in one basket," Hill had a different opinion. He believed that concentrated attention to one purpose is the best way to achieve it. Where there is a plan A, B, and C, the focus is split in many directions, and so are our energies. A backup plan, in that regard, can be ineffectual. I realized that everything that I have ever done successfully has happened because I put all my focus and energy into that goal.

A heart attack can be a powerful wake-up call. Healing requires the development of a one-track mind about getting better and improving your quality of life. Every day should move you one step closer to fulfilling that purpose.

Next, it's essential to know where you are going. Like driving a car, we go from point A to point B. When we get into a car, we typically don't drive aimlessly. And, if we need to take a detour and become lost, we find a map, or turn on our navigation, to help us find the way back on track. In working with the goal of good health, it's best to create a roadmap or plan of action—which Hill's concepts provide—to take the quickest route forward.

Support

It is completely natural to be scared and depressed, after suffering a heart attack or any major life threatening illness, as we discussed in Chapter Seven. We need support. Reach out and ask for it. Don't just sit at home and be afraid, do something, you are still alive.

Some of us may be too proud to ask for help, but that position dilutes the power of the goal. My father was too proud to get help outside the family. We might judge that pride as being blind to his very need for good health, but it's important to remember that, in the 1970s and 1980s, support groups and cardiac rehab units were less common. Today, we have more options.

Reach out for support. When you do, I believe that the right person will come to your aid. There are many people who are willing and lovingly ready to help you. It was hard for me to ask for help, too. I'm used to being the one taking care of everyone else, doing all the research, and being of service for others. Now, like me, it's your turn to ask for help. Find a support group, get private counseling, go to cardiac rehab—do whatever it takes to get back in life again.

If you're reading this book, you have survived your heart attack—or maybe even more than one. My point is that you're still alive—not yet dead. I encourage you to engage with life and begin to live fully again.

Hill connects the need for support to what he calls our "mastermind alliance." A mastermind alliance is a group of two or more people committed to achieving a specific *goal*. We all have mastermind alliances. You have one with your spouse or partner. You have one with your doctor or health care team. After I determined my goal of heart healing and decided to get the support, I looked for my mastermind alliance. I chose a person that I knew had my best interests at heart and was willing to go the extra mile for me. This person became my research partner and, as I described in Chapter Five, helped me with the research that I needed to do. She helped me to avoid the feelings of depression and vulnerability that overwhelmed me when I tried reading research about women and heart attacks alone.

When we begin to enlist help, we also begin to overcome our fears and start developing our positive mental attitude. We do this by learning enough to develop informed opinions and knowledge about heart disease *and* how it relates to us as individuals.

Although I am more than capable of doing this work on my own, after my heart attacks, my psyche was susceptible to suggestion by what doctors and researchers had to say. I became mentally vulnerable due to my physically weakened condition. I needed my research partner, my mastermind, to help me sort through all of their opinions and agendas.

Today, I understand that research into heart disease isn't an exact science. For each study, there is a population of people chosen, and these people—often called "samples"—cannot represent everyone and everyone's circumstances. That's why I eventually felt comfortable enough telling my doctors that I did see myself as a unique individual who could affect her own health. Research represents a fraction of the population, which means there is considerable bias. We need to account in research for gender, ethnicity, and cultural environment, just to name a few populations, which is why we need to develop critical thinking about our illnesses and health potential. People who are our support system can help with this major task.

Applying Faith

Faith is a belief or trust in someone or something. Some think of faith as religious faith, something bigger than ourselves, something omnipresent, God, the universe. I think of faith as belief. The power of faith is so immense that we can do anything if we simply believe we can.

To apply faith, in Hill's context, means to act. Faith in action is applied faith. Without action, without doing something about our health, nothing positive can happen. However, applied faith doesn't always mean physical action because action can come in the forms of meditation, positive thinking, and prayer. Applied faith is a state of mind where we release control and allow God or our Higher Power to help us. I believe this level of applied faith is essential for healing.

In learning to change our health circumstances, it's also critical to become fearless. Hill teaches us that faith and fear simply cannot coexist. Even if we start out with some fear, we can take that fear and act anyway. When we move forward in faith, we move despite any fear and the fear eventually dissipates.

How can we build and strengthen faith? The first step is overcome the disbelief in our minds. Let go of:

- ❤ Worrisome thoughts.

- ❤ Statements that begin with I don't have enough…

- ❤ Anger of poor health.

- ❤ Fear of changing.

- ❤ Any other negative thought.

<u>After releasing these negative thoughts, try this three-step plan</u>:

1. Identify your purpose. Back up this purpose with desire. To ignite your desire, link it to a motive like returning to health and well-being.

2. Decide how you are going to achieve step one. Make a plan.

3. Put that plan into action. Nothing ever happens if you don't begin.

Applied faith can be as simple and as meaningful as a prayer of gratitude, where thankfulness for all the blessing in life is given. To maintain the good health that I have gained, I say a prayer of gratitude in the morning and at night. In the Bible's book of Matthew (17:20), Jesus said: "I tell you the truth. If you have faith as small as a mustard seed, you can say to this mountain, 'Move from here to there' and it will move. Nothing will be impossible for you." Like all seeds, the seeds of faith in our ability to become healthy must be cultivated to grow. Prayer applies the action for faith to become reality.

Using These Principles to Gain Sound Health

To develop sound mental and physical health, we must consider the body/mind/spirit connection. In fact, for sound health, it is critical to understand the body/mind/spirit as inseparable; they work together and for each other. Without this understanding, any effort toward good health simply is a Band-Aid solution.

Positive Mental Attitude

To develop sound mental health, you must condition your mind, like an athlete training for the Olympics. Your sound mental health toolkit might contain the following type of affirmation:

Positive mental attitude says I CAN. I know that only I can control my own mind. After my heart attack, I was in shock and disbelief, but then I became grateful and realized that I had learned about my sick heart in time to do something about it. I now have the ability to change directions and make positive improvements. To have a positive mental attitude, I am clearing my mind of any negativity. My positive mental attitude is my first step to healing.

Here is a formula for attaining and using a positive mental attitude. Apply this rule: **R³A=PMA**.

- ❤ Positive Mental Attitude—A positive mind says I CAN.

- ❤ Recognize—Only you can control your own mind.

- ❤ Realize—There is something to be gleaned from this experience.

♥ Resolution—Clear your mind of negativity so that only positive thoughts reside.

♥ Action—Apply action to what you want, start where you are, and do it now.

Self-Discipline

Self-discipline is necessary to control your mind. Just try holding a thought for one minute. Try doing it now. Hold the thought. What happened? Did you think of something else? Did other thoughts drift in? Most likely, the answer is yes. Most of us cannot control one minute of thinking, which means that we need a great deal of self-discipline in all areas of our lives—time, our emotions, our appetites, and mental attitude.

Time is something we cannot accrue. There is only a limited amount of time. We can't make more time in the same way we can make more money. We must control and manage our time, wisely. Think quality when thinking about time. There are only twenty-four hours in a day. How will we manage it? You have eight hours to sleep, eight hours to work, and eight hours left for you. However, many people are stuck in traffic, some for two-to-four hours a day just commuting. That doesn't seem to be an appropriate use of time. What do you do for yourself and your family every day? What do you do for pleasure? Write down what you do with your time. Like a money budget, make yourself a time budget.

Emotions control our state of mind. After a heart attack, emotions are tenuous. We may feel like we are on the outside looking in at life. We are scared because we aren't sure whether life will return to normal again, and we had a close brush with death. It may take some time to heal our emotions. What I had to do was find my happy place, which was buying and caring for horses. These actions returned me to a time of carefree happiness. Nonetheless, I had to retrain my brain to remember those happy times. Find things that make you happy. It could be connecting with nature, drawing or painting. Learn to control your emotions by changing them. When emotions are attached to a thought, your subconscious mind will act. It is like a child acting out the mirror image of his or her parents.

Appetite is something we all need to control, me included. I love food. However, a stomach is only as big as a fist. Eat to live; don't live to eat. Appetite doesn't involve only food, however. Appetite includes other things or substances that are harmful, such as drinking excessive alcohol, using recreational drugs, and smoking. It amazes me how many people still smoke after a heart attack. Some need a few attacks before it sinks in that they should stop. If you smoke, please stop. Essentially, when you smoke you are deep breathing for at least ten minutes. Start doing deep breathing instead of grabbing a smoke, and remember that self-discipline controls your mind.

Here is a formula for attaining and using self-discipline. Apply this rule: **C⁴TEAM=SD.**

- ♥ Self-Discipline—Control your mind.

- ♥ Time—Control and manage time. Use it wisely because you cannot make more of it.

- ♥ Emotions—Control your emotions and your state of mind.

- ♥ Appetite—Control your appetite, food, drinking, and smoking.

- ♥ Mental Attitude—Control your mental attitude through PMA.

Accurate Thinking

Accurate thinking is extremely crucial to healing. But when we are sick, it often is hard to think accurately. Nonetheless, the most important question to ask is: *How do I know this information is correct?* I ask this question all the time. Especially in medical situations, we must learn how to differentiate information that is important and not important to separate fact from fiction, and to distinguish experts from non-experts. When I started doing my heart health research, I was surprised to learn that many of the publications seven years ago didn't have good heart protocols for women and, in fact, most of the studies focused on men. I told my doctors that the medication they prescribed was studied on men, not women. We had to compromise on my medication regimen.

Here is a formula for attaining and using accurate thinking. Apply this rule: $D^3INFO^2=AT$.

- ❤ Accurate Thinking—Ask how you know this information is correct.

- ❤ Differentiate the Important from what is NOT important.

- ❤ Differentiate Fact from fiction.

- ❤ Differentiate Opinions from experts or non-experts.

Personal Initiative

Personal initiative is necessary for healing to occur because there's no way around the fact that heart healing requires action on our part. First, we need to have a plan to know the direction we are going. For example, if the goal is to start healing the heart, we should write a plan. What are the first steps? For me, it was to start charting my daily actions and symptoms because I needed to find out what my problem was so I could prevent the next attack.

Here is a formula for attaining and using personal initiative. Apply this rule: **ASK=PI.**

- ❤ Personal Initiative — Take action for healing to occur.

- ❤ Ability to act — And go the extra mile.

- ❤ Self-starter — Many can start, but only a handful will finish.

- ❤ Know where you are going — Have a goal and a plan.

Adversity and Defeat

When adversity or defeat happens, do you look at the world as hopeful or hopeless? Both adversity and defeat can be a blessing in disguise. Crisis has two meanings:

- ❤ A sense of catastrophe or peril

- ❤ A sense of available opportunity

There is always possibility, but sometimes we can't see it at the time of the adversity. Often, we can't see the opportunity until we look back over the past. Here, you may wonder what the blessing is in having a heart attack. Frankly, I started by being grateful that I survived. I saw the heart attacks as signals to change direction in my life. By surviving a heart attack, we have a second chance to make lifestyle changes, slow down, take a self-inventory, and focus on what is right and good in life. We need to take action to help ourselves, but again sometimes, we need a helping hand.

Here is a formula for making the most of adversity and defeat. Apply this rule: **BLESSING=AD.**

Adversity and **D**efeat — There is always a silver lining.

Brother's keeper — Anything that hurts you hurts everyone around you. Please realize that people around you are hurting too.

- ❤ Learning from defeat — Is your glass half full or half empty?

- ❤ Equivalent seed of benefit — Crisis has two meanings, one of which is an opportunity.

- ❤ Spend time counting your gains — Rather than your losses.

- ❤ Stop, look, and listen — Take inventory of yourself after this wakeup call.

- ❤ Important moment when you realize defeat — Now you are ready for change.

- ❤ No such thing as permanent defeat — Whether you achieve success or failure is up to you.

- ❤ Germination — You have been given a seed that requires cultivation.

Going the Extra Mile

Going the extra mile is the sibling of personal initiative. Normally, we make this kind of effort in the work place. We reap what we sow in life. The quality and quantity of service that we can give with a positive mental attitude is what going the extra mile is all about. How does this point relate to heart health?

Sometimes, it's hard for people to do this hard work for themselves. If you are struggling and can't believe in yourself at this time, take yourself out of the picture and insert your own child or your inner child. We know that we will go to extraordinary lengths to help our children. We have to love ourselves that much, too. We will go above, and beyond the call of duty when it comes to our children. We will find out all we can, we will learn, we will take action to bring about a change for our children. This kind of effort is what we must do for ourselves, too.

Here is a formula for going the extra mile. Apply this rule: Q^2 **ESP =GEM**

❤ Going the Extra Mile is related to taking personal initiative.

❤ Quantity and Quality of service given — We reap what we sow.

❤ Excellent Service with a PMA.

Figure 8.3: Components of Sound Health

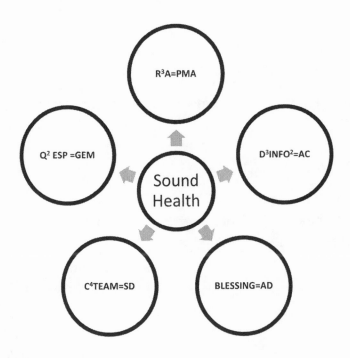

Your Heart-Mind

As I said earlier, there are two types of heart patients: one who wants to get well and has a positive mental attitude, and one who wants to get well but has a negative mental attitude. The first type of patient — through effort, determination, and will power — may be able to heal herself fully or partially. The difference is an intention to heal. Frankly, I don't believe that we can heal fully without this focused intentionality.

The body/mind/spirit connection is extraordinarily powerful. In many ways, though, the mind controls the body. Like a computer, the mind is the operating system that directs the hardware, which is the body. However, the heart has its own brain, so to speak, which shares common molecules and signaling pathways with the brain. In fact, neuroscientists now know that it's possible to change the brain by training the mind to promote positive brain changes through social and emotional learning.

When you have a heart attack, it's an emotional event that involves emotional learning. The brain perceives a threat or danger and reacts with fear. Fear causes more stress on the heart. This perceived threat can make some people believe that every pain experienced is associated with their heart. Many heart patients feel this way. I had the same experience the first year. I became afraid to do anything, and every pain made me more concerned about my heart.

Another example is that of phantom shocks. I have spoken to many patients with implanted defibrillators. Once the defibrillator has gone off, some people will develop what is known as "phantom shocks." They tell me that they are experiencing shocks, but their doctors and electrophysiologists can't find any evidence. They are so afraid of being shocked that they are gripped with fear. They are so terrified of getting shocked that this increases their stress level to the point of needing medication just to cope. To them, the shocks are real and frightening.

Such phenomena aren't new. In fact, before doctors implanted heart devices, my father experienced extreme fear of getting cardioversion, which was a shock-induced correction of atrial fibrillation (AF). The shock corrected the arrhythmia by resynchronizing his heart. He was so fearful of being shocked that it was painful to watch him stress over it. Each time he needed the treatment, his fear grew worse. My point is that our brains have the ability to change for both better and worse. This ability is known as *neuroplasticity.*

The heart is the seat of all emotions; it sends messages to the brain, and the brain instructs the body. This is why it's necessary to clear your heart of emotions when you're intending to get well from a heart attack. I know you may feel sad, angry, and scared. In your heart, you may be holding fear, which is translated through the brain's pathways. Imagine that when the brain receives the fear signal, a cascading effect of signals moves throughout the body and causes more stress on the heart.

Deep Breathing to Heart Health

To prevent this additional stress on the heart, it's important to discharge any negative emotions you're keeping in it. One way to do this is through deep breathing exercises that help to release all the tension in your body. Another way is to employ the power of forgiveness. Forgive yourself for being sick in the first place, and forgive your heart for having "attacked" your body. Instead, love and cherish your heart so that it will send positive waves of healing throughout your body.

As I worked to heal my heart, I started deep breathing exercises while in bed at night. At first, I don't think I could get past seven breaths before I started sobbing. It was a cathartic release of emotional pain and fear. If you have a similar experience, think of it as cleaning house and de-cluttering. I was careful to control this cleansing experience so that I was not overly emotional. I did this deep breathing exercise each night until I felt peace and could do it without crying.

Meditation to Heart Health

After the deep breathing exercise, I started a meditation using several of the affirmations listed below:

- ❤ I am getter better and better each and every day.

- ❤ No one can make me upset or work me up.

- ❤ I am happy; I am whole.

- ❤ My heart is beautiful. It pumps blood freely throughout my veins and arteries.

- ❤ My heart is perfect, and it has the perfect shape.

- ❤ My heart is powerful and has healed itself.

- ❤ My heart is amazing.

- ❤ My heart beats easily and effortlessly.

- ❤ My heart signals other cells if it needs help.

- ❤ My heart knows how to heal itself, and it does so easily.

- ❤ Every day, I am getting stronger and even better than before.

- ❤ I make healthy eating choices. [Substitute smoking or sleeping or exercise or other word choices that fit your situation.]

In this type of affirmative meditation, you send a message to your subconscious mind. Such messaging is a way of programming yourself to good health. As Hill said, *"what the mind of man can conceive and believe, it can achieve."* I prefer this one, *"what the mind can conceive and believe, the body can achieve."* This is your ABC's to Achieve, you must Believe and Conceive.

Now, I meditate every night before I go to sleep. It's crucial to get sound rest in healing, and meditation is one way to get that rest. Meditation is so powerful that it can help to condition the mind to begin the healing process. The injured heart needs the same kind of care as a child. So, during the most crucial months of healing, I also practiced ten-to-fifteen minutes of meditation throughout the day.

Here is another meditation that you can practice *as is* or modify to meet your individual needs:

Close your eyes and imagine that, in your heart-mind, there is a child – your child. Take a few deep breaths, focusing on the child of your heart. Maybe you will see a baby or young child. She smells heavenly as you take her into your arms. Tell her that everything is going to be all right. Comfort her. Love her. Hold her close. Ask for forgiveness. Tell her that you will never leave her. You will always protect and watch over her.

Some people will do more for their children than they will for themselves. For example, as a mother, you exercise some self-discipline around your child (or baby). You don't give your child a diet of soft drinks and candy. No! You give the child healthy foods. You make sure she gets good nutritious food, exercise, rest, and intellectual stimulation. You treat your child well. In the same way, if your heart-mind holds your child, you will treat your heart-mind well, too.

It takes about twenty-one days for a habit to become second nature. One way to build a habit of meditation is to modify the affirmations and meditations that I provided above to make them your own. Record it with your own voice and listen to it twice a day. I know you will begin to feel better and start to experience peace of mind.

Music to Heal the Heart

Another strategy for healing my heart-mind is to play music that is reminiscent of happy years. When I was healing my heart, I listened to songs that raised happy memories and emotions. This practice filled me with joy, which is positive for my brain and, thus, for my heart's healing. Art, dancing, and writing creatively also can help to discover and develop these pleasant memories.

Identifying What I Want

We can get what we want only if we identify it first. Without identifying our heart's desire and body's needs, we can't attain them. Ask yourself these questions:

What do you want?

I want _____ .

What do you need to get it?

*I need*_____ .

What is keeping you for getting it?

_____ is keeping me from getting it.

Use your responses to these questions to signal necessary changes in your life.

Changing My Beliefs

Let's look at your belief system. After you have had a heart attack, your beliefs may sound like this:

I'm a heart patient.

I'm sick.

My heart is weak.

My heart has been damaged.

I'm a ticking time bomb. (Sadly, this was father's favorite expression.)

These are the dominant negative suggestions that we give ourselves. When we say these things and our families repeat or agree with them, we reinforce the negative and false belief system of being sick.

Let's try again.

I'm **not** a heart patient.

I'm **not** sick.

My heart is **not** weak.

My heart has **not** been damaged.

I'm **not** a ticking time bomb.

Notice the words _**not**_ and _**never**_. The subconscious mind can disregard presence of negative words like **_couldn't, wouldn't, shouldn't, can't, no, not,_** and **_never,_** for example. By saying the above statements — even with _not_ and _never_ in them, you're reinforcing the disease in your body because the mind can disregard the negative words.

What you are really saying is:

I'm a heart patient.

I'm sick.

My heart is weak.

My heart has been damaged.

I'm a ticking time bomb.

See the difference?

At first, I also thought of myself as a heart patient, but I had to stop that kind of negative thinking. I asked my family not to refer to me as a heart patient, too. I turned these negative statements into positive statements that affirmed good health by reframing the negative sentences with positive words. For example, I said these positive things:

- ❤ I'm healthy.

- ❤ I'm well.

- ❤ My heart is strong.

- ❤ My heart is healthy.

- ❤ My heart is perfect.

- ❤ I'm getting stronger each and every day.

- ❤ I'm returning to full health.

Now create your own positive sentences. Remember to avoid the negative statements that include *not* and *never*; instead, use positive phrases that say the good things about you and your health that you intend to have happen. It may be difficult to do at first because 90% of the self talk we do is negative. Now you try:

I am _____

My heart is _____

_____

_____

_____

_____

Acting Healthy to Heal the Heart

Healthy people not only think healthy thoughts, but they also act in healthy ways that send a positive message to the body.

For example, sitting on the couch afraid to do anything reinforces a sense of being sick. Healthy actions include:

- ♥ If you cannot drive, have someone drive you to the park or sit outside in your garden. Look for something to focus on and appreciate the beauty of it.

- ♥ Take long walks, and be happy to be present in the moment. This behavior reinforces wellness and rebuilds strength.

- ♥ Go to cardiac rehab, if possible, to learn realistic limitations and how to move into better health. I didn't have that option, so I always had people around me or not too far away. They made sure I wasn't alone in case of another possible heart attack, and they also provided much-needed emotional support.

A Healthy Mind for a Healthy Heart

Hill once said, "If you think you are sick, you are."

In order to achieve healing after a heart attack, the body/mind/spirit connection must be recognized. Our mental attitudes are keys to our success. I understand that it's difficult to be positive after a heart attack. I was scared and waiting for the next heart attack. I had to take that fear and turn its negative energy around to motivate me positively. I decided to surround myself only with positive people and significantly limited my contact with negative people. I worked hard to reframe everything I experienced in positive ways.

What's so positive about having a heart attack? That's a good question, so let's use it as an example:

- ♥ First, you can be happy you are alive!

- ♥ You can be thankful that you have a second chance to do anything and everything you want to do.

- ❤ You can be appreciative to all the people involved in your wonderful health care.

- ❤ You can be a beacon to help others and give back some of your good fortune.

- ❤ You can change your lifestyle to be happier, healthy, and positive.

- ❤ You can start to love yourself more and more every day.

- ❤ You can forgive yourself and others — improving your life and theirs.

- ❤ You can say and do things for and with your family, making peace and leaving regret behind.

A heart attack can be a blessing in disguise. It forces us to slow down and see all the things in life for which we have to be grateful. Without such a wake-up call, everyday hustle and bustle can make us too busy and lead to unhealthy cynicism. When we are so busy, we act as if we don't have time for anything — even to get better! This negative way of life does not need to be our reality. The heart attack can lead to recovery not only in body, but also in mind and spirit when we take advantage of the changes it calls for. We need only to slow down and take time to breathe and appreciate life and all its many blessings.

Lessons Learned

1. The foundations for healing from a heart attack or other heart disease are found within us in our body/mind/spirit connection. The key is to have a positive mental attitude and to chase away negativity with thought patterns and actions that promote good health.

2. We need to set an intention to heal with a goal of perfect heart health. This intention to heal requires the support of others who can believe in our goals. Faith in God or a higher power allows us to move away from fear and to put our goals into action.

3. The strong body/mind/spirit connection means that what happens in our hearts — both emotionally and physically — can be shaped by our minds and spirits. Techniques for conquering fear and developing a positive mental attitude toward healing our hearts include:

   a) Deep breathing exercises.

   b) Mediation.

   c) Using music and other sensory stimulation that promotes peace and joy to stimulate healing.

   d) Identifying what we want in order to get what we need.

   e) Changing negative beliefs.

   f) Acting healthy to become healthy.

   g) Developing a healthy mind and spirit.

PART THREE

THE WAY FORWARD

NINE
CHAPTER

Collaborative Approach to Healing from Heart Disease

O
ne of the goals of this book is to encourage readers to create a health care team that works for each of us individually. Although some medical centers and doctors attempt to create such a collaborative team for us, many of us will have to do that important work on our own. I include this brief chapter in Part Three because I believe this is a new direction that heart patients — with their advocates — may need to forge both during healing years and afterwards as they maintain their health.

In a recent research project for my Masters of Science (MSc.) in Clinical Research, I learned that a patient's quality of life is impacted by many different factors. Most important for our needs as heart attack survivors, a patients' quality of life may be improved significantly by using a multidisciplinary team approach, which represents a patient-centered focus on the part of health care providers.

Patient quality of life is a significant factor in healing and in the development of new approaches to heart health—such as that of autologous stem cell (ASC) treatments, which I mentioned in the Introduction and discuss further in Chapter Ten. In some cases, proving that a treatment leads to an improved quality of life is important because it may encourage the U. S. Food and Drug Administration (FDA) to approve alternative heart treatments including stem cell treatments. Until the FDA approves stem cells as an alternative treatment, it won't be available in the U. S., and American patients will continue to travel to other countries to receive it.

Quality of life is a perception about our physical and mental health over a period of time, and that perception is based on our values, goals, expectations, standards, and concerns (CDC, 2010a; WHO, 1997b; JAMA, 2002). The idea of quality of life is complex because extrinsic life-changing factors can affect our physical health and psychological state. Two characteristics of quality of life are "objective functioning and subjective well-being" (Muldoon et al., 1998). These characteristics evaluate the impact of illness and treatment relative to daily life activities and life satisfaction. Objective functioning measures the patient's physical well-being and functional ability, whereas subjective well-being measures emotional and social well-being (Cella, 1994).

Quality of life is an essential component of determining whether a treatment is effective. Some patients believe that their quality of life is more important than their quantity or length of life, as a recent study funded by the European Commission indicated. The PRIMSA group and Kings College London conducted a telephone survey of 9,344 respondents. The study addressed European respondents' preference for quality of life versus quantity of life from seven countries: England, Belgium, Germany, Italy, Netherlands, Spain, and Portugal. The survey asked respondents about their priorities when faced with a life-threatening disease with limited time to live: 71% wanted to improve their quality of life, whereas only 4% thought both quality of life and health were equally valuable (BMJ Blogs, 2011a; King College London, 2011). In fact, according to Nicolau (cited in Shipper, 1983), "quality of life is a critical factor in determining survival." Patients want to know the benefits of the treatment regardless of its scientific value. On the other hand, some patients may opt to decline treatment due to the poor quality of life caused by the treatment itself.

Research supports that a multidisciplinary team approach improves patient outcome with some treatments (Rich et al., 1995). From subjective experience with patients, researchers know that patient attitude is critical to regaining health or having a sense of wellbeing (Sears et al., 2004). Optimistic patients typically have had a positive improvement on quality of life measurements, such as better mental health and social functioning (Sears et al.), whereas patients with negative beliefs appear to be more susceptible to depression and decreased quality of life (Hallas et al., 2010). In fact, negative emotions like anger, anxiety, and depression are risk factors for coronary heart disease (Kubzansky & Kawachi, 2000), as I have shown in this book.

Such experiences strongly suggest that the medical community needs to consider a holistic approach to patient care. A multidisciplinary team can offer a holistic and patient-centered approach to patient care by providing support and counseling and by encouraging patients and families to adopt healthy lifestyles. The team also can implement tailored programs to prepare patients for their treatments. The major change that such a team presents is that it would be patient-centered rather than provider-centered.

In the future, my hope is that all of us will experience a paradigm shift, where we become active participants in our health care. I think that patients like you and I need to take charge of our heath care by developing—hiring, firing, and coordinating—our own health care teams when the medical facility or doctors can't or won't do this for us.

A multidisciplinary team is a collaboration of health professionals. For example, a cardiovascular multidisciplinary team may include:

- ❤ A patient coordinator to serve as the liaison
- ❤ An experienced cardiovascular research nurse
- ❤ A registered dietitian
- ❤ A social service professional
- ❤ A counselor
- ❤ A cardiologist
- ❤ Follow up services offered by a variety of health care providers

The multidisciplinary team for ASC transplant, for example, works in collaboration with patients to educate, facilitate pre-transplant and post-transplant care, and to provide follow-up care. Any multidisciplinary team establishes a critical layer of communication among patients and their physicians. The team alerts the physicians to valuable insights regarding patients and helps develop treatment plans. Such an approach is patient-centered in its attention to patients' overall responses to the medical treatment, as opposed to the clinically discernible responses alone. A carefully orchestrated timing of events among the team and the patients contributes to what I call the Patient Collaborative Experience®, which sits within the Chain of Health® model. In the model below all patients will fit regardless of their current health status. This innovative process that I have developed is focused on prevention programs and getting people back into a state of health. The processes are complex but this is just a birds-eye view. The Chain of Health® model will be piloted in Europe, within the next five years.

Figure 9.1: Chain of Health

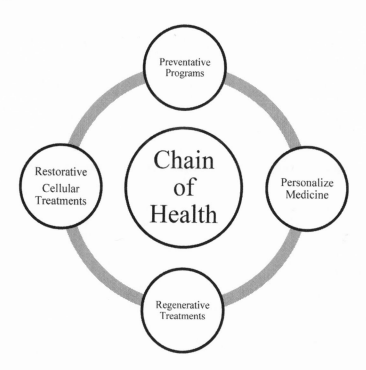

In my professional experience, patients supported by a Patient Collaborative Experience® expressed that, they felt more supported, calmer, healthier, and more positive overall. Others health care professionals have expressed similar experiences. For example, Boutron et al. (1995) reported that some patients said they felt well enough for early discharge, which is advantageous from the perspective of reducing costs alone. Multidisciplinary team leaders develop full optimization plans prior to treatment and post treatment. If, for example, a patient needs to lose weight or quit smoking, a team is formulated to help her achieve her health goals.

Where I work, the Patient Collaborative Experience® model has been practiced by our patient care coordinators since 2005. Patients receive care coordination, patient education, resource identification, and whatever else they require. Patient navigators/coordinators play a pivotal role in helping patients traverse a complex continuum (Campbell et al., 2010). The Patient Collaborative Experience® model should be used for patient care more broadly than just going to your doctor when there is a problem. Although this process would be the best choice, however, where it doesn't exist, we have to forge the trail for ourselves.

Medical professionals have often questioned why some patients have exceptional results while others have slight-to-moderate improvement after treatment for heart failure. In some patients, an underlying psychological factor appears to be involved. Pedersen et al. (2010) suggested that patients with Type D (distressed) personality have an impact on their heart failure outcomes because they conceal a high degree of emotional distress. It seems likely that such patients' outcomes could be significantly improved by using a Patient Collaborative Experience® approach where their emotional needs are addressed.

When patients have few options and everything that traditional medicine can do has been done, they may seek alternatives measures. Patients need someone who can talk with them about their concerns and questions when they seek complementary or novel treatments. Adding an extra layer of care such as a patient coordinator to a collaborative team could be especially useful.

Sadly, there are many patients who are afraid to communicate with their cardiologists, fearing even to ask for their records or to get a second opinion. Many patients do not want their cardiologist to know they are researching alternative treatments. It is critical, though, to keep the cardiologist informed and in the loop. Unfortunately, many patients find that when they present new information to their doctors, the doctors are not receptive. In fact, many have expressed that they were humiliated, intimidated, berated, and others were simply afraid of being ostracized or discharged as patients. For the most part, patients want to improve their quality of life. I think that improved quality of life can occur with a multidisciplinary team approach for all patients because some of this necessary receptivity is built into the health care.

To this end, I urge you to consider which health care professionals you need and want in your team. Then, assemble this team approach with your doctors. If you cannot persuade your cardiologist or other primary doctor to take an approach that you believe will improve your quality of life, then decide whether you want to stay with this doctor. There is a fine line here and you need to make sure that you do not alienate yourself, therefore, you must be diplomatic at all times. If you do stay, then you may need to develop the team on your own.

Perhaps the simplest way of doing so is to stay within one medical center's network. There are well-regarded medical centers in most urban communities and in some suburban ones, as well. The doctors who connect with these centers tend to know each other and will communicate fairly freely. Their medical notes are probably available through a standardized computer network, making your job of seeing complementary providers much easier.

However, it also is possible to create a multidisciplinary team among geographically dispersed medical and health care providers. One couple I know sees physicians both at Duke University in North Carolina and the National Institutes of Health in Washington, D. C. The doctors work together with the Duke physicians taking the lead. In any multidisciplinary team approach, one doctor may be the team leader. Usually, it will be the cardiologist that you most often see or the specialist that treats your specific heart disease. You may need to be more involved in assisting the doctors with sharing information in this scenario, but you can build in many of the same quality of life measures for your personal care.

Advocate for yourself to get the best medical care possible. Self-advocacy is critical to becoming healthy again. You and your heart deserve it!

TEN

CHAPTER

Life After A Heart Attack

Heart attacks change lives. They change our family's lives, our friends' lives, and—most of all—they change our own lives.

In the early days after my first heart attack, I was stunned and felt as if I had lost control of my body. I quickly changed my eating habits, but then had two more heart attacks anyway. Not only were they worse than the first, but my doctors remained puzzled as to why I had them. After charting my symptoms, taking my medications, researching heart disease and supplementation, talking with specialists and others who could support me—in other words, after taking care of my body/mind/spirit—I began to get a handle on what had happened to me. And, my healthy activities and positive mental attitude have led to healing myself to the extent that my heart no longer shows any evidence of damage, for all intents and purposes, I'm healed and well. I still do everything to keep myself healthy, and that includes seeing my doctor on a regular basis.

Is there life after a heart attack? Yes. This chapter illustrates how my life has changed for the better, which at first I could not have imagined, sometimes you have step back to put things in perspective. My prayer is that you, too, will find such a rewarding life.

Autologous Stem Cell Research

In Chapter Three, I said that Dad's situation was why I didn't wait to seek alternative (novel) treatments. Months after my heart attacks, I learned about autologous stem cell (ASC) research for heart therapy. I wanted to be proactive and sought stem cell treatment to heal any damage I had sustained with my heart attacks. I was determined not to follow the path of "wait and see" with medication that didn't seem right for me.

Stem cell research has been a contentious issue in the news, so it's important to know that ASCs come from our own cells. Because these cells are not embryonic and not harvested from unknown people, there isn't a highly charged ethical debate around their use. With ASC, my own cells could make me healthy.

I was very interested in this type of medicine for two reasons. First, I thought of my father and how he was a pioneer as an early transplant recipient. I thought about how stem cells might have benefited him prior to his transplant. Perhaps with stem cells he might have avoided the heart transplant or possibly might have kept his own heart long enough for medicine to advance. Second, I thought of myself and of all the other women who would prefer use their own cells to heal their hearts rather than to have a coronary artery bypass graph.

From my research, I became thrilled that I didn't have a stent. Although after the second angiogram I was disappointed, because there was no diagnosis and without it there could be no prognosis. I was relieved not to have a stent after I learned that it is only a temporary solution, and that, within five years, most patients need bypass surgery. In the meantime, having a stent means being on drugs permanently to prevent blood clots. Although I didn't have either procedure, because my coronary arteries were normal, I wanted to know whether stem cells could help heal my heart and reverse any damage or scar tissue.

In November 2005, Kurt and I traveled overseas to investigate a stem cell company that uses ASC derived from peripheral blood. We visited the hospitals, and we met the doctors and owners of the company that was conducting the research. I was more than impressed with the entire approach from the time of arrival to the time of departure. A patient would receive first-class, concierge service all the way.

The doctors impressed me as highly intelligent and thoughtful, and they gave me excellent advice. One tidbit that I gleaned from one of the cardiologists was to be careful lifting anything heavy, which made perfect sense. When we pick-up something heavy without doing any aerobic exercise before the lift, the blood pressure can spike, or rise sharply. This spike in blood pressure can cause a piece of plaque to dislodge and create a blockage, which could lead to a heart attack. His caution included a ban on shoveling snow and doing any type of heavy lifting like moving furniture. I was surprised that no one had ever told me these things before. Perhaps I would have learned such practical tips had cardiac rehab been available.

The doctor also explained the importance of heart safety, which was to have the heart rate and blood pressure rise at the same time, rather than for the blood pressure to rise by itself. This physician was highly regarded and a physician to royalty. He ordered a perfusion test, called a sestamibi stress test or MIBI for short. After the results of this test and others, he congratulated me: "You are the first person I've met to have 100% perfusion. You don't need stem cells!" I was impressed. The company easily could have taken advantage of my desire for wellness and taken my money, but they didn't. They absolutely refused to accept me into the stem cell program.

They offered me a job instead!

A New Career

Today, I am a consultant for biotech companies, and a clinical researcher with a special interest in autologous stem cells and its cardiovascular applications. One organization impressed me to such an extent that I felt honored to speak with their cardiovascular patients and educate them on using their own cells to help heal their bodies. I truly understand their fears because of my father's history, the work I did in helping to organize his transplant team, and my personal heart health story.

When patients have no options and everything that traditional medicine can do has been done, they may seek alternatives measures. When seeking alternative treatments such as experimental ASC, patients want the trusted advice of their physicians. However, ten minutes with a physician is considered a long visit from the physician's perspective and yet too little time to make a decision on stem cell treatments — or any treatment, for that matter. In fact, many patients tell me that they are lucky to get only three minutes after waiting for thirty-to-sixty minutes. For this reason, when I'm not working for the stem cell research company, I work as a consultant, where cardiac stem cell patients can inquire about treatment and get honest answers in a realistic timeframe.

I remember speaking to one man who was from the Middle East. I sensed that he believed I couldn't possibly know how he felt. He seemed to be thinking: *What does she know?* Normally, when I work with inquiring stem cell patients, I avoid talking about myself unless it seems beneficial. The conversation is about that person — not me. But in this instance, I said, "You know, you probably think I have no idea what you feel or that I don't know anything, but you are wrong."

I told him that I had suffered three heart attacks and that I understood his fears.

Every pain you feel — it doesn't matter where it's coming from — you immediately think, "Oh, my heavens; it's my heart or it must be related somehow to my heart." You have an impending sense of doom. You wonder if you are going to die today. You think to yourself that you could drop dead at any moment. No one cares. You don't want to do anything. You're afraid to be alone. You are awake, but you are not actually living. You're so crippled with fear that you're afraid to do anything. You think no one understands what you're going through. Then, you try to justify everything, and you start experiencing grief — denying what has happened, being angry at the world, and wonder why is this happening to me.

Pretty soon, I could hear him starting to chuckle, his chuckle then turning into laughter. He said: "You are right! That is exactly how I feel, and I cannot talk to anyone because no one understands."

I know many of you readers can relate to his feelings. We've all been there, as Chapter Seven described.

Do you really need stem cells? Maybe. Maybe not. I didn't need them, and I healed myself with the measures described in this book.

However, I have witnessed dramatic transformations with some people. One woman only wanted to be able to pick up her grandson. Her cardiologist tried to convince her not to come for treatment and tried to intimidate her with thoughts of hepatitis and AIDS. Despite her cardiologist, she came for ASC treatment. For her, the treatment was a miracle, which makes my job all the more rewarding. She is off the transplant list, and her ejection fraction is above 50%, which she attributes to stem cell therapy. She has her life back and can now pick up her grandson. Five years later, she remains healthy.

Recently, I worked with a man who has a two-year old son. His cardiologist recommended that he have a defibrillator implanted. He was scared and didn't want it if his ejection fraction could improve. He decided to have ASC treatments. As a result, his ejection fraction increased by 65% post treatment. When his cardiologist asked him what had happened, he replied that he'd had the stem cell treatment. His doctor replied that he had stabilized his heart and no longer needed a defibrillator. Since that time, he has transformed his life by losing weight and living differently. His health brings me joy to be in a new career. Today, nearly a year later, his ejection fraction is almost normal, and the couple is expecting their second child!

I find great joy in the many benefits I see in people who have experienced healing through ASC and subsequently changed their lifestyles. Sadly, there are some people for whom stem cell treatments have not helped. There are several reasons for these results — many physical in nature. I often wonder if some patients actually reach a point of diminishing return. In other words, why wait until you are so weakened to have ASC treatment? Some patients are proactive, and some are reactive. Proactive patients come at once, whereas, reactive patients come when they have experienced a setback, i.e. ejection fraction decrease.

I do think, however, that people who have experienced better health after ASC and other heart-related therapies tend to have a mindset similar to that of a winning athlete. These people want to live, and they optimize their lives with positive thinking, healthy and fresh food. In addition, they quit smoking, lose weight, and deal with emotional issues. Not everyone who qualifies needs stem cells. I remember getting a phone call from a woman whose heart was too large for a heart sleeve clinical trial. She excitedly told me that she no longer needed stem cells. When I asked what she had done to produce this new result, she said, "I did what you did." Her doctor was shocked at her significant improvement although he neither confirmed nor denied that what she was doing was the reason for her new found recovery. He only said, "Whatever you are doing, keep doing it."

Many people have reported the same kind of improvement. If people are dying from heart disease—especially women, who are the heretofore ignored gender—and want to live, I certainly will tell them what I did to heal myself. That's what this book is all about.

Coming Full Circle

I'm a firm believer that life's lessons repeat themselves until we learn something from them. Prior to my heart attacks, I was pondering what my life was all about and how I could leave my footprint in the world. I felt alone since my career in Norway was derailed.

After I healed my heart and began working for a biotech cellular company, I was in the kitchen and suddenly a thought popped into my mind: I had now come full circle and returned to medicine in my life and career. I said to Kurt, "Isn't it funny how life is?"

He replied, "What do you mean?"

I said, "Well, I had to have these heart attacks, which led me to learn how find healing in my heart, which finally led me to ASC work and back into medicine!"

During this time, I decided to take on a second master's degree, an MSc in Clinical Research that I earned in 2011. I really enjoy research and want to make a difference in the area of ASC. If I never had the heart attacks, I would never have returned to school, found lifesaving ASC for cardiovascular patients, or written this book to help all of you.

Thank you for listening to my story. My wish for you is healing and good health. I would love to hear from you and your stories. You can reach me through http://www.dorinaerbo.com

APPENDIX A

Quit Smoking Script

Read this script into a recorder. Set your pace so that it takes about thirty minutes to read. Listen to the recording every day for at least twenty-one days, and then listen once a week for reinforcement. **Do not listen to this script while driving or operating any machinery.** *Get into a relaxed position like one of the following:*

- ❤ *Sitting in a chair with legs uncrossed and both feet on the floor. Close your eyes and relax your hands.*

- ❤ *Sitting cross-legged on the floor in a classic meditative position. Relax your hands on your knees in an open, palms-up position.*

- ❤ *Lying on your back with arms and legs relaxed. Use a pillow under your legs to flatten your back.*

SCRIPT

I take a nice, deep breath. I breathe all the way in past my lungs and into my abdomen. Then, I exhale slowly, releasing all tension and worries as I breathe out. Again, I take a nice, deep breath, all the way in, and exhale slowly, releasing all tension and cares.

I'm aware of any sounds that I may hear, and I realize that those sounds simply are life going on. I bring my attention and thoughts inside the room and into my own body.

Breathing slowly and deeply, I'm relaxing and becoming more and more comfortable. I'm just melting and feeling comfortable, just letting all my cares drift away.

As I take another deep breath, I exhale all the cares and any worries I have right now. Each and every breath I take sends a wave of relaxation all the way from the top of my head down to the tip of my toes. I become more and more relaxed with each and every breath I take.

The more relaxed I become, the deeper I go into myself.

I know that smoking is a poison to my body. I need my body to be healthy so I can enjoy life to its fullest in every way. I'm now learning to respect my body.

As I become more deeply aware and in tune with my body with each and every breath I take, I become more and more relaxed. The more relaxed I become, the deeper I go into myself.

In my mind's eye, I imagine the most beautiful, peaceful place, a place that holds meaning for me. I may hear some familiar sounds or smell familiar aromas. I feel a sense of harmony and peace around me.

Now, I let all the muscles in my face relax.

I'm experiencing a beautiful, relaxed, natural feeling in my body.

Now, I imagine myself at home sitting where I normally sit and relax and smoke a lot. I see this happening. At the same time, I'm aware of the beautiful, relaxed, natural feeling I have in my body right now.

As I experience the beautiful, relaxed, natural feeling in my body, I imagine myself begin to reach for a pack of cigarettes, as I have done so many times in the past.

As I hold the pack up in my hands, I feel the shiny, smooth texture of the cellophane on my fingertips, the corners of the pack in the palm of my hand. I even smell the tobacco through the cellophane.

I'm aware of the beautiful, relaxed, natural feeling I have in my body right now.

At this moment, I make up my mind to be a non-smoker permanently!

I take the pack of cigarettes and squeeze them in my hand. And I THROW them DOWN on the floor. I watch them BOUNCE and ROLL OVER as I STEP on them.

I'm enjoying stomping and crushing the box. I feel the pressure going down my leg to my foot as I'm SQUEEZING, SQUASHING, and GRINDING those cigarettes right into the floor.

As I step back from those cigarettes, I notice that the cellophane is torn off the package, the package is FLATTENED and CRUSHED, and the tobacco is coming through the torn paper. I REALIZE the POWER I have over those cigarettes.

They are just lying there on the ground. They are not talking back, fighting back, or yelling back. They are just lying there like the nothing that they are, and I realize the power I have over those cigarettes.

I now take control over my mind and body, and I like that.

I take those cigarettes and kick them with my foot, and they go up into the air and end up in the trash completely out of my sight.

And just as those cigarettes disappeared from my sight, any desire for a cigarette now and at any time in the future dissolves and dissipates from my mind.

Each and every time I read or hear a recording of this script, I see myself as a non-smoker with a sense of pride—feeling free, clean, and healthy.

I have now kicked the habit! I'm free! I'm a non-smoker by my choice!

I have eliminated over 1,200 toxic ingredients from my mind, my body, my environment, and the environment of my family and my loved ones.

Now that I'm a non-smoker by my choice, each and every breath I bring into my lungs is filled natural air and loaded with healthy oxygen. That oxygen is going to every cell, tissue, and muscle fiber of my body all the way down to my toes and out to my fingertips.

I now have more energy and vitality than I have had in a long, long time! And my mind is clear. I'm now adding life to my living and living to my life.

After all, I came into this world as a non-smoker, and now with the power and the ability of my conscious and subconscious mind, I choose to return to my natural and normal state permanently.

I remember a time during elementary (primary) school when I was a non-smoker. I imagine the buildings and playgrounds of my school. It's recess time. I watch myself on the playground with my childhood friends and classmates. Some of them are talking, laughing, screaming, and playing. These are all the typical things I would hear and see during recess time at my elementary school.

I see myself as a non-smoker. I see myself as a non-smoker, going home from school, clean and healthy.

After all, I came into the world as a non-smoker, and I now choose to return to that normal, natural state, permanently!

This will be the easiest and the smoothest transition I have ever made to an important goal, and it's permanent!

I remember the first cigarette I ever smoked. I remember clearly how bad it was. It was hot and burning in my lungs. I had to learn to smoke. Anything that I have learned, I can change. I can unlearn it, and I know that. Stored in my conscious and subconscious mind is my memory of being a non-smoker. I now choose to return to that normal, natural state permanently!

This will be the easiest and most permanent transition I have ever made to an important goal. I have stopped smoking, and it's permanent!

Now, I remember a time when I was confronted with challenge, and I met that challenge, and I felt really good about myself. I had a sense of pride, a sense of accomplishment—I remember that time and feeling so well.

I hold that feeling of pride and sense of accomplishment. If at any time in the future I realize that I want a cigarette—and I doubt that I will, but if I do—I'll say silently and inwardly: I'M FREE. With those words, I'll feel healthy and in control. I'll tell myself that I'm healthy and in control.

My keywords are: "I'm free." When I say my keywords "I'm free," that same feeling of pride and sense of accomplishment emerges in my body. That feeling is so strong that the desire for cigarettes leaves me entirely.

I repeat my keywords: "I'm free! I'm free! I'm free! I'm free! I'm free!"

Anytime I hear the word "non-smoker," I think of myself as a non-smoker. I feel the same sense of pride and accomplishment as I do with the words "I'm free." I'm truly on the right track.

Now, I imagine that I'm around others who may be smoking—I may be out socially, or I may be at their home. But I continue to see myself as a non-smoker.

Other people can smoke if they want to, but I see myself as a non-smoker. All of my life, I have seen smokers and non-smokers mixing and mingling, but one has no effect on the other. Now I choose to be the non-smoker. Congratulations!

Now that I'm a non-smoker, my nose is more sensitive to the traces of formaldehyde and ammonia in cigarette smoke, and I realize that I'm truly on the right track.

Now when I take a shower, my clothes, my hair, my body, and my breath remain fresh longer. And I like that! I see myself as a non-smoker and what it means to me. I realize I'm truly on the right track.

Now, I see myself driving in my car as a non-smoker and appreciating the fresh air. I see myself at home as a non-smoker—calm, cool, and relaxed, totally in charge of my mind and my body. I see myself around others who may be smoking, but I see myself as a non-smoker.

I'm a non-smoker by choice, and my taste buds are coming alive. I'm able to taste the intricate and subtle differences in food and flavors. Small portions of food satisfy me completely. I take into my body only those foods that are nutritionally good for me. I see myself as slim, trim, firm, at my ideal weight—and a non-smoker.

Now, I go back to my special place in my mind's eye, the most beautiful, peaceful place, a place that holds meaning for me. I may hear some familiar sounds or smell some familiar aromas. I feel a sense of harmony and peace around me.

I feel the relaxation in my body, going down to my toes and fingertips, totally experiencing the beautiful, relaxed, natural feelings in my body.

As I concentrate on that beautiful, peaceful, serene place, I take deep breath—all the way in. As I exhale, I bring my thumb and index finger together and rub them gently and continue to rub them as I speak.

Anytime I feel tight, nervous, or tense, or if I have a desire for a cigarette, my thumb and index finger automatically will come together and a wave of relaxation will go right through my body, and I'll feel as good as I do right now.

I'll now separate my thumb and index finger. As my hand relaxes, I feel myself going deeper and deeper into relaxation.

My body knows that smoking is a poison. I cannot live without my body. I owe my precious body respect and protection. Being a non-smoker is my way of acknowledging the precious nature of my body and at the same time, my way of seeing me as my body's keeper.

Now that I have made this commitment to respect my body, I have within me the power to have smoked my last cigarette. Congratulations!

It feels so good to be smoke-free—to be in control of my life—no longer allowing dangerous, destructive habits to control me.

Every day as a non-smoker, my self-confidence, self-esteem, and self-respect grow deeper and deeper.

It feels so great to be able to breathe better, have more energy, and feel happy about myself.

The feeling and emotion of love is the strongest emotion that humans have, and with that feeling, I can accomplish anything. I feel the love that I have in my relationships and the love I have for others who are around me, and I realize that I'm cleaning up the environment. I serve as an inspiration for others.

I know how much being a non-smoker means to my family. They love me, and I love them. They want me to live and continue to be around for a long time. They want me to continue to play an active part in their lives.

My family and my continued relationships with them are more important than smoking.

I feel good about myself and my commitment to be a non-smoker. I'm truly on the right track.

Now I'm going to count up from one to five. At the count of five, I'll allow the energy and vitality to return to my mind and body. I'll feel as though I've had one or two hours of deep, relaxing energizing sleep.

- ❤ <u>One</u> — I'm beginning to return to energy and vitality.

- ❤ <u>Two</u> — I'm feeling the relaxation in my body knowing that I'm a new person and a winner. I can accomplish anything I set my mind to, and I have complete confidence in my abilities as a non-smoker.

- ❤ <u>Three</u> — I see myself as a non-smoker, with a sense of pride, a sense of accomplishment, and feeling clean and healthy.

- ❤ <u>Four</u> — I take a deep breath, bringing in all the vital life-giving oxygen. I bring in that energy and vitality and, as I exhale, I let anything negative flow out of my mind. My mind is now full of positive expectancy.

- ❤ <u>Five</u> — Now I'm fully aware once again, feeling invigorated, refreshed, and relaxed. I take a deep breath, stretch, and get ready to continue my day.

APPENDIX B

Weight Loss Script

Read this script into a recorder. Set your pace so that it takes about thirty minutes to read. Listen to the recording every day for at least twenty-one days, and then listen once a week for reinforcement. **Do not listen to this script while driving or operating any machinery.** *Get into a relaxed position like one of the following:*

- ❤ *Sitting in a chair with legs uncrossed and both feet on the floor. Close your eyes and relax your hands.*

- ❤ *Sitting cross-legged on the floor in a classic meditative position. Relax your hands on your knees in an open, palms-up position.*

- ❤ *Lying on your back with arms and legs relaxed. Use a pillow under your legs to get comfortable.*

SCRIPT

I take a nice, deep breath. I breathe all the way in past my lungs and into my abdomen. Then, I exhale slowly, releasing all tension and worries as I breathe out. Again, I take a nice, deep breath, all the way in, and exhale slowly, releasing all tension and cares.

I'm aware of any sounds that I may hear, and I realize that those sounds simply are just life going on. I bring my attention and thoughts inside the room and into my own body.

Breathing slowly and deeply, I'm relaxing and becoming more and more comfortable. I'm just melting and feeling comfortable, just letting all my cares drift away.

As I take another deep breath, I exhale all the cares and any worries I have right now. Each and every breath I take sends a wave of relaxation all the way from the top of my head down to the tip of my toes. I become more and more relaxed with each and every breath I take.

The more relaxed I become, the deeper I go into myself.

I now visualize my body and the weight I want to be. I see myself at that weight now. I feel great at this new weight. I see myself as calm and self-confident and full of self-love. I see myself as thin.

I'm at peace with my own feelings. I'm safe where I'm right now. I create my own security. I love and approve of myself. I create my life the way I want it to be.

I only eat when I'm physically hungry. When I'm upset or worried or angry or sad, food is unappealing. I only eat when I'm physically hungry.

Each and every bite that I take allows my taste buds to savor the flavor of the good and healthy foods I eat. With each bite I take, I put the fork down to rest between bites. As I put down the fork, I notice the size of my fist. I realize that my stomach is only the size of my fist. My stomach is so small.

I now plan my meals. When I shop for food, I make a list. When I shop for food, I shop on a full stomach. When I shop for food, I shop along the walls of the store because that is where the healthiest and freshest food is located. I stay away from the center aisles because that is where all the processed foods are. I buy fresh and healthy food instead of foods that are processed. Whenever possible, I avoid food that is in a package, box, bottle, or can.

I need and want only those foods that are good for my body.

I always sit while eating. When I'm at home, I eat in the dining room or at a table in the kitchen area.

I enjoy drinking water. It's very cool and refreshing, and I like the taste. I find myself thirstier than I ever was before. Now that I'm eating well, I'm drinking more water. Every day I drink at least six to eight glasses of water. I avoid alcohol or drink it very sparingly if I drink it at all.

Staying on this eating program is simple and easy. I'm at peace with my feelings. I'm safe where I am. I create my own security. I love and approve of myself. I now create my own life the way I want it to be.

My body is becoming smaller and getting smaller with every day that passes. My clothes fit better, and I feel healthier.

I remember that stuffy feeling I had after I used to eat those big holiday dinners. I begin to feel that stuffy feeling, now. I visualize my stomach as small and full.

As soon as I feel that stuffy feeling, I stop eating. I'm full. I stop. That stuffy feeling is a signal that my body gives me to let me know that I have had enough. When I have had enough, I stop eating. My stomach is small and requires less food than I used to eat.

Since I now love and respect my body, I listen to its signals. I respond appropriately by stopping. I listen to my body when it feels full. In turn, when I think "thin," my body begins to metabolize fat.

I am enjoying a new eating habit. I always lay my knife and fork down between bites, and I think only of the bite that is in my mouth.

I'm enjoying a new tasting habit. Because I think only of the bite that is in my mouth, I enjoy the taste of it much more. My taste buds become more sensitive, and I get more satisfaction from each bite.

I eat slowly, I need much less, and I enjoy it more. When I see something that I would like to taste — perhaps a dessert — it's okay to take a taste. A taste means one or two bites, which is just enough to satisfy my curiosity.

Now I'm aware of the visual appeal of the food, the way it looks, the aroma of the food, the way it smells, and the way it feels in my mouth. I taste and savor the flavor. My taste buds become thoroughly satisfied in just taking one or two bites.

After I have taken one or two bites, I'm perfectly satisfied in every way. I put the fork or spoon down on the plate, and I walk away feeling completely satisfied in every way.

Staying on this eating program is simple and easy. I'm at peace with my feelings. I'm safe where I am. I create my own security. I love and approve of myself. I now create my own life the way I want it to be.

My goal is to lose three pounds of this ugly, unwanted fat each week. I now imagine three 16-ounce raw steaks tied around my body. I throw away this much weight each week, and my body looks and feels much better.

I begin an exercise program. The more I exercise, the better I feel, and the better I feel, the more I exercise.

I'm looking better and feeling better. My clothes are fitting loosely.

I feel good about myself. I find myself smiling more and walking differently. Everyone is noticing how good I look.

❤ I respect my body.

❤ I choose a healthy life.

❤ I respect my body.

❤ When I think of my body, I think thin.

❤ I think thin.

❤ I become thin.

❤ I am thin.

❤ I respect my body.

Now I'm going to count up from one to five. At the count of five, I'll allow the energy and vitality to return to my mind and body. I'll feel as though I have had one to two hours of deep, relaxing energizing sleep.

❤ One—I'm beginning to return to energy and vitality.

❤ Two—I'm feeling the relaxation in my body knowing that I'm a new person and a winner. And I can accomplish anything I set my mind to. I have great confidence in my abilities as a person who is eating smaller portions and losing weight.

❤ Three—I see myself as a thinner and healthier person with a sense of pride, a sense of accomplishment, and feeling whole and healthy.

❤ Four—I take a deep breath, bringing in all the vital life-giving oxygen. I bring in that energy and vitality and, as I exhale, I let anything negative flow out of my mind. My mind is now full of positive expectancy.

❤ Five—Now I'm fully aware once again, feeling invigorated, refreshed, and relaxed. I take a deep breath, stretch, and get ready to continue my day.

APPENDIX C

Symptoms and Medication Chart

Date:			(Red Flags)	
Observations:				
Time	Dosage	Description (Medication, OTC, Daily Intake)	Home Measures (Blood pressure, pulse, glucose)	Nitro/ Period

Date:				(Red Flags)	
Observations:					
Time	Dosage	Description (Medication, OTC, Daily Intake)		Home Measures (Blood pressure, pulse, glucose)	Nitro/ Period

APPENDIX C

Date:			(Red Flags)		
Observations:					
Time	**Dosage**	**Description (Medication, OTC, Daily Intake)**	**Home Measures (Blood pressure, pulse, glucose)**		**Nitro/ Period**

APPENDIX D

Symptoms Chart Using SOAP

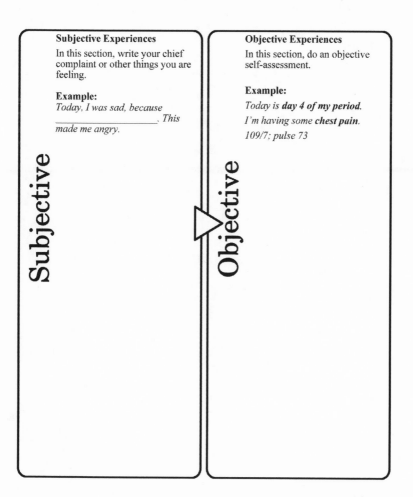

Subjective Experiences

In this section, write your chief complaint or other things you are feeling.

Example:
Today, I was sad, because
_____. *This made me angry.*

Subjective

Objective Experiences

In this section, do an objective self-assessment.

Example:
*Today is **day 4 of my period**.*
*I'm having some **chest pain**.*
109/7; pulse 73

Objective

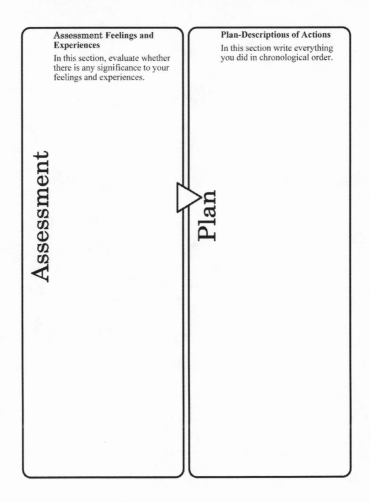

Assessment Feelings and Experiences

In this section, evaluate whether there is any significance to your feelings and experiences.

Plan-Descriptions of Actions

In this section write everything you did in chronological order.

Assessment

Plan

APPENDIX E

BMI Chart

See next page

A Height (Ft.in., Meter)	C Body Mass Index = BMI	Normal BMI 18.5 - 24.9						Overweight BMI 25 - 29.9					Obese BMI 30 and above					
	B Body Weight (Pounds, KG, and Stones)	19	20	21	22	23	24	25	26	27	28	29	30	31	32	33	34	35
4'10" (58") 1.47		91	96	100	105	110	115	119	124	129	134	138	143	148	153	158	162	167
		41.3	43.5	45.4	47.6	49.9	52.2	54	56.2	58.5	60.8	62.6	64.9	67.1	69.4	71.7	73.5	75.7
		6.5	6.85	7.14	63.5	7.85	8.21	8.5	8.85	9.21	9.57	9.85	10.21	10.57	10.92	11.28	11.57	11.92
4'11" (59") 1.50		94	99	104	109	114	119	124	128	133	138	143	148	153	158	163	168	173
		42.6	44.9	47.2	49.4	51.7	54	56.2	58.1	60.3	62.6	64.9	67.1	69.4	71.7	73.9	76.2	78.5
		6.71	7.07	7.42	7.78	8.14	8.5	8.85	9.14	9.5	9.85	10.21	10.57	10.92	11.28	11.64	12	12.35
5'0" (60") 1.52		97	102	107	112	118	123	128	133	138	143	148	153	158	163	168	174	179
		44	46.3	48.5	50.8	53.5	55.8	58.1	60.3	62.6	64.9	67.1	69.4	71.7	73.9	76.2	76.2	81.2
		6.92	7.28	7.64	8	8.42	8.78	9.14	9.5	9.85	10.21	10.57	10.92	11.28	11.64	12	12.42	12.78
5'1" (61") 1.55		100	106	111	116	122	127	132	137	143	148	153	158	164	169	174	180	185
		45.4	48.1	50.3	52.6	55.3	57.6	59.9	62.1	64.9	67.1	69.4	71.7	74.4	76.7	76.2	81.6	83.9
		7.14	7.57	7.92	8.28	8.71	9.07	9.42	9.78	10.21	10.57	10.92	11.28	11.71	12.07	12.42	12.85	13.21
5'2" (62") 1.57		104	109	115	120	126	131	136	142	147	153	158	164	169	175	180	186	191
		47.2	49.4	52.2	54.4	57.2	59.4	61.7	64.4	66.7	69.4	71.7	74.4	76.7	79.4	81.6	84.4	86.6
		7.42	7.78	8.21	8.57	9	9.35	9.71	10.14	10.5	10.92	11.28	11.71	12.07	12.5	12.85	13.28	13.64
5'3" (63") 1.60		107	113	118	124	130	135	141	146	152	158	163	169	175	180	186	191	197
		48.5	51.3	53.5	56.2	59	61.2	64	66.2	68.9	71.7	73.9	76.7	79.4	81.6	84.4	86.6	89.4
		7.64	8.07	8.42	8.85	9.28	9.64	10.07	10.42	10.85	11.28	11.64	12.07	12.5	12.85	13.28	13.64	14.07

Appendix E

A Height (Ft.in., Meter)

C Body Mass Index = BMI

B Body Weight (Pounds, KG, and Stones)

Height	Measure	Normal BMI 18.5 - 24.9						Overweight 2 5 - 2 9. 9						Normal BMI 18.5 - 24.9 Obese 30 and above					
	BMI	19	20	21	22	23	24	25	26	27	28	29	30	31	32	33	34	35
5'4" (64") 1.63	Pounds	110	116	122	128	134	140	145	151	157	163	169	171	180	186	192	197	204
	KG	49.9	52.6	55.3	58.1	60.8	63.5	65.8	68.5	71.2	73.9	76.7	77.6	81.6	84.4	87.1	89.4	92.5
	Stones	7.85	8.28	8.71	9.14	9.57	10	10.35	10.78	11.21	11.64	12.07	12.21	12.85	13.28	13.71	14.07	14.57
5'5" (65") 1.65	Pounds	114	120	126	132	138	144	150	156	162	168	174	180	186	192	198	204	210
	KG	51.7	54.4	57.2	59.9	62.6	65.3	68	70.8	73.5	76.2	78.9	81.6	84.4	87.1	89.8	92.5	95.3
	Stones	8.14	8.57	9	9.42	9.85	10.28	10.71	11.14	11.57	12	12.42	12.85	13.28	13.71	14.14	14.57	15
5'6" (66") 1.68	Pounds	118	124	130	136	142	148	155	161	167	173	179	186	192	198	204	210	216
	KG	53.5	56.2	59	61.7	64.4	67.1	70.3	73	75.7	78.5	81.2	84.4	87.1	89.8	92.5	95.3	98
	Stones	8.42	8.85	9.28	9.71	10.14	10.57	11.07	11.5	11.92	12.35	12.78	13.28	13.71	14.14	14.57	15	15.42
5'7" (67") 1.7	Pounds	121	127	134	140	146	153	159	166	172	178	185	191	198	204	211	217	223
	KG	54.9	57.6	60.8	63.5	66.2	69.4	72.1	75.3	78	80.7	83.9	86.6	89.8	92.5	95.7	98.4	101
	Stones	8.64	9.07	9.57	10	10.42	10.92	11.35	11.85	12.28	12.71	13.21	13.64	14.14	14.57	15.07	15.5	15.92
5'8" (68") 1.73	Pounds	125	131	138	144	151	158	164	171	177	184	190	197	203	210	216	223	230
	KG	56.7	59.4	62.6	65.3	68.5	71.7	74.4	77.6	80.3	83.5	86.2	89.4	86.2	95.3	98	101	104
	Stones	8.92	9.35	9.85	10.28	10.78	11.28	11.71	12.21	12.64	13.14	13.57	14.07	14.5	15	15.42	15.92	16.42
5'9" (69") 1.75	Pounds	128	135	142	149	155	162	169	176	182	189	196	203	209	216	223	230	236
	KG	58.1	61.2	64.4	67.6	70.3	73.5	76.7	79.8	82.6	85.7	88.9	92.1	94.8	98	101	104	107
	Stones	9.14	9.64	10.14	10.64	11.07	11.57	12.07	12.57	13	13.5	14	14.5	14.92	15.42	15.92	16.42	16.85

A Height (Ft.in., Meter)	C Body Mass Index = BMI																
	Normal BMI 18.5 - 24.9						Overweight 25 - 29.9					Normal BMI 18.5 - 24.9 Obese 30 and above					
	19	20	21	22	23	24	25	26	27	28	29	30	31	32	33	34	35
B Body Weight (Pounds, KG, and Stones)																	
5'10" (70") 1.78	132 / 59.9 / 9.42	139 / 63 / 9.92	146 / 66.2 / 10.42	153 / 69.4 / 10.92	160 / 72.6 / 11.42	167 / 75.7 / 11.92	174 / 78.9 / 12.42	181 / 82.1 / 12.92	188 / 85.3 / 13.42	195 / 88.5 / 13.92	202 / 91.6 / 14.42	209 / 94.8 / 14.92	216 / 98 / 15.42	222 / 101 / 15.85	229 / 104 / 16.35	236 / 107 / 16.85	243 / 110 / 17.35
5'11" (71") 1.8	136 / 61.7 / 9.71	143 / 64.9 / 10.21	150 / 68 / 10.71	157 / 71.2 / 11.21	165 / 74.8 / 11.78	172 / 78 / 12.28	179 / 81.2 / 12.78	186 / 84.4 / 13.28	193 / 87.5 / 13.78	200 / 90.7 / 14.28	208 / 94.3 / 14.85	215 / 97.5 / 15.35	222 / 101 / 15.85	229 / 104 / 16.35	236 / 107 / 16.85	243 / 110 / 17.35	250 / 113 / 17.85
6'1" (73") 1.85	144 / 65.3 / 10.28	151 / 68.5 / 10.78	159 / 72.1 / 11.35	166 / 75.3 / 11.85	174 / 78.9 / 12.42	182 / 82.6 / 13	189 / 85.7 / 13.5	197 / 89.4 / 14.07	204 / 92.5 / 14.57	212 / 96.2 / 15.14	219 / 99.3 / 15.64	227 / 103 / 16.21	235 / 103 / 16.78	242 / 110 / 17.28	250 / 113 / 17.85	257 / 117 / 18.35	265 / 120 / 18.92
6'2" (74") 1.88	148 / 67.1 / 10.57	155 / 70.3 / 11.07	163 / 73.9 / 11.64	171 / 77.6 / 12.21	179 / 81.2 / 12.78	186 / 84.4 / 13.28	197 / 89.4 / 14.07	202 / 91.6 / 14.42	210 / 95.3 / 15	218 / 98.9 / 14.42	225 / 102 / 16.07	233 / 106 / 16.64	241 / 109 / 17.21	249 / 113 / 17.78	256 / 116 / 18.28	264 / 120 / 18.85	272 / 123 / 19.42
6'3" (75") 1.91	152 / 68.9 / 10.85	160 / 72.6 / 11.42	168 / 76.2 / 12	176 / 79.8 / 12.57	184 / 83.5 / 13.14	192 / 87.1 / 13.71	200 / 90.7 / 14.28	208 / 94.3 / 14.85	216 / 94.3 / 15.42	224 / 102 / 16	232 / 105 / 16.57	240 / 63.5 / 17.14	248 / 112 / 17.71	256 / 116 / 18.28	264 / 120 / 18.85	272 / 123 / 19.42	297 / 135 / 21.21

APPENDIX F

Napoleon Hill
Seventeen Principles

In the *Science of Success*, Napoleon Hill describes seventeen principles. Principle 15, the *Maintenance of Sound Health* encompasses and uses several of the other principles.

The Seventeen Principles

1. Definiteness of Purpose
2. The Mastermind Alliance
3. Applied Faith
4. Go the Extra Mile
5. Pleasing Personality
6. Personal Initiative
7. Positive Mental Attitude
8. Enthusiasm
9. Self Discipline
10. Accurate Thinking
11. Controlled Attention
12. Teamwork
13. Learning from Adversity and Defeat
14. Creative Vision
15. Maintenance of Sound Health
16. Budget Time and Money
17. Cosmic Habitforce

These principles work in conjunction with one another. The principles that I used in my self-healing are bolded in black. The beauty of Hill's principles is that we cannot enact one principle without engaging other principles. Throughout this book, I have engaged all these principles, which I believe are essential to a heart attack patient's recovery to good health.

Definiteness of Purpose 1

Master Mind 2

Applied Faith 3

Going the Extra Mile 4

Pleasing Personality 5

Personal Initiative 6

Positive Mental Attitude 7

• **Definiteness of Purpose 1 , Master Mind 2, Applied Faith 3, Sound Heath 15**

Enthusiasm 8

Self Discipline 9

Accurate Thinking 10

Controlled Attention 11

Teamwork 12

Adversity and Defeat 13

Creative Vision 14

Sound Heath 15

• **PMA 7, Self Discipline 9 ,Accurate Thinking 10, Personal Initiative 6, Learning from Adversity and Defeat 13, Going the Extra Mile 4**

Time and Money 16

Cosmic Habitforce 17

REFERENCES

American Heart Association. (2011). 1994 Revisions to classification of functional capacity and objective assessment of patients with diseases of the heart. Retrieved from: http://www.american-heart.org/presenter.jhtml?identifier=1712

Anderson, J. L., Adams, C. D., Antman, E. M., Bridges, C. R., Califf, R. M., Casey, Jr, D. E., Chavey II, W. E., ... & Wright, R. S. (2011). ACCF/AHA focused update incorporated into the ACC/AHA 2007 guidelines for the management of patients with unstable angina/non-STelevation myocardial infarction: a report of the American College of Cardiology Foundation/American Heart Association Task Force on Practice Guidelines. *Journal of the American College of Cardiology, 57,* 215-367. doi: 10.1161/CIR.0b013e318212bb8b

Arom K. V., Ruengsakulrach, P., & Jotisakulratana, V. (2008). Intramyocardial angiogenic cell precursor injection for cardiomyopathy. *Asian Cardiovascular Thoracic Annual, 16,* 143-148 Retrieved from http://asianannals.ctsnetjournals.org/cgi/reprint/16/2/143?maxtoshow=&hits=10&RESULTFORMAT=&author1=Arom&andorexactfulltext=and&searchid=1&FIRSTINDEX=0&sortspec=relevance&resourcetype=HWCIT (Accessed: 14 February 2011).

Arom, K. V., Ruengsakulrach, P., Belkin, B., & Tiensuwan, M. (2009). Intramyocardial angiogenic cell precursors in non-ischemic dilated cardiomyopathy. *Asian Cardiovascular Thoracic Annual, 17,* 382 - 388. Retrieved from http://asianannals.

ctsnetjournals.org/cgi/content/full/17/4/382?maxtoshow=
&hits=10&RESULTFORMAT=&author1=Arom&andorexactf
ulltext=and&searchid=1&FIRSTINDEX=0&sortspec=relevan
ce&resourcetype=HWCIT

Assmus, B., Schächinger, V., Teupe, C., Britten, M., Lehmann, R., Döbert, N., ... & Zeiher, A. M. (2002). Transplantation of progenitor cells and regeneration enhancement in acute myocardial infarction. *TOPCARE-AMI*, Circulation 106, 3009-3017. Retrieved from http://circ.ahajournals.org/cgi/reprint/106/24/3009

Bairey Merz, C. N., Johnson, B., Delia, S., Barry L., Bittner, V., Berga, S. L., Braunstein, G. D., ... & Sopko, G. (2003). Hypoestrogenemia of hypothalamic origin and coronary artery disease in premenopausal women: A report from the NHLBI-sponsored WISE study. *Journal of American College of Cardiology, 41*: 413-419

Beeken, R. J., Eiser, C., & Dalley. C. (2010). Health-related quality of life in haematopoietic stem cell transplant survivors: a qualitative study on the role of psychosocial variables and response shifts. *Quality of Life Research.* doi: 10.1007/s11136-010-9737-y

BMJ Blogs. (2010). Comet initiative. (Blog). Retrieved from http://blogs.bmj.com/bmj/2010/03/08/the-comet-initiative/

BMJ Blogs. (2011). 'Quality' more important than 'quantity' at end of life. (Blog). Retrieved from http://blogs.bmj.com/spcare/2011/03/29/individuals-place-greater-value-on-quality-than-quantity-at-end-of-life/

Brown, M. S. (1990). *U. S. Patent No. 4 933 165*. Washington, DC: U. S. Patent and Trademark Office.

Bundkirchen, A. & Schwinger, R. H. G. (2004). Epidemiology and economic burden of chronic heart failure. *European Heart Journal Supplement, 6*, D57-D60. doi:10.1016/j.ehjsup.2004.05.015

Burg, M. M. & Abrams, D. (2001). Depression in chronic medical illness: The case of coronary heart disease. *Journal of Clinical Psychology, 57,* 1323–1337. doi: 10.1002/jclp.1100

Campbell, C., Craig, J., Eggert, J., & Bailey-Dorton, C. (2010). Implementing and measuring the impact of patient navigation at a comprehensive community cancer center. *Oncology Nursing Forum, 37*(1). [Online]. Available from: http://www.metapress.com.ezproxy.liv.ac.uk/content/n213np7n3x147344/

Canadian Cardiovascular Society. (2011). Canadian Cardiovascular Society grading of angina pectoris. Retrieved from http://www.ccs.ca/download/position_statements/Grading%20of%20Angina.pdf

Cao, G., Alession, H. M., & Cutler, R. G. (1993). Oxygen-radical absorbance capacity assay for antioxidants. *Free Radical Biology and Medicine, 14*: 303–311.

Cao, G., Verdon, C.P., Wu A. H., Wang, H., & Prior, R. L. (1995). Automated assay of oxygen radical absorbance capacity with the COBAS FARA II. *Clinical Chemistry, 14*(12 Pt 1):1738-44.

Cardiovascular Outcomes, Inc. (2011). The Kansas City cardiomyopathy questionnaire. Retrieved from http://cvoutcomes.org/topics/3038

Cella, D. F. (1994). Quality of life: Concepts and definition. *Journal of Pain and Symptom Management, 9*(3), 186-192. doi: 10.1016/0885-3924(94)90129-5

Center for Disease Control. (2010). About CDC. Retrieved from http://www.cdc.gov/about/

Center for Disease Control. (2010). Health related quality of life. Retrieved from http://www.cdc.gov/hrqol/

Center for Disease Control. (2010). Heart disease facts. Retrieved from http://www.cdc.gov/heartdisease/facts.htm

Center for Disease Control. (2001). Diabetes and women's health across the life stages: A public health perspective. Retrieved from http://www.cdc.gov/diabetes/pubs/women/index. htm

Center for Disease Control & National Center for Health Statistics. (2007). Leading causes of death by age group, all females United States. Retrieved from http://www.cdc.gov/women/lcod/archive/index.htm

Christian, A. H., Rosamond, W., & White, A. R., Mosca, L. (2007). Nine-year trends and racial and ethnic disparities in women's awareness of CHD and stroke: An American Heart Association national study. *Journal of Women's Health, 16,* 68-81.

Claassen, J. (2005). The gold standard: Not a golden standard. *British Medical Journal, 330,* 1121. Retrieved from http://www.bmj.com/content/330/7500/1121.full#cited-by

Coyne, K. S., & Allen, J. K. (1998). Assessment of functional status in patients with cardiac disease. *Heart & Lung: The Journal of Acute and Critical Care, 27*(4), 263-273. Retrieved from http://www.sciencedirect.com/science?_ob=MImg&_imagekey=B6WG74CNT29H431&_cdi=6815&_user=8554888&_pii=S0147956398900383&_origin=search&_zone=rslt_list_item&_coverDate=08%2F31%2F1998&_sk=999729995&wchp=dGLzVlb-zSkzV&md5=ebbed0cf6c688c8730e2bcd7f4c2fa05&ie=/sdarticle.pdf

Creswell, J. (2003). Research design: Qualitative, quantitative, and mixed methods approaches. New York, NY: Sage Publications, Inc.

Doering, L. V. & Eastwood, J. A. (2011). A Literature review of depression, anxiety, and cardiovascular disease in women. *Journal of Obstetric, Gynecologic, & Neonatal Nursing, 40*(348), 361. doi: 10.1111/j.1552-6909.2011.01236.x

Donald, A. (2003). What is Quality of Life? [Online].http://www. whatisthisseries.co.uk Accessed 30 November 2010.

Edelson, E. (2005). Brain Damage Is Linked to Heart Failure. Brain Institute Research, UCLA. Retrieved from http://www.bri. ucla.edu/bri_weekly/news_050822.asp

Folkers, K., Langsjoen, P. H., Willis, R., Richardson P., Xia L., Ye C., & Tamagawa, H. (1990). Lovastatin decreases coenzyme Q levels in humans. *Proceedings of the National Academy of Sciences, 87,* 8931-8934.

Folkers, K., Vadhanavikit, S., Mortensen S. A. (1985). Biochemical rationale and myocardial tissue data on the effective therapy of cardiomyopathy with coenzyme Q10. *Proceedings of the National Academy of Sciences, 82*(3), 901-904.

Franceschini, N., Rose, K. M., Storti, K. L., Rutherford, S., Voruganti, V. S., Laston, S., Göring, H. H. H., ... & North, K. E. (2009). Social- and behavioral-specific genetic effects on blood pressure traits: The strong heart family study. *Circulation Cardiovascular Genetics,* 2:396-401; doi:10.1161/CIRCGENET-ICS.109.853630

Friedman, M. & Rosenman, R. H. (1974). *Type A behavior and your heart.* New York: Knopf.

Gazzaniga, D. A., Fowler, M. B., & Gazzaniga-Moloo, J., (2001). *The no-salt, lowest-sodium cookbook.* New York: St. Martin's Press.

Gibbons, R. J., Abrams, J., Chatterjee, K., Daley, J., Deedwania, P. C., Douglas, J. S., Ferguson, T. B. Jr., ... & Smith, S. C. Jr. (2003). ACC/AHA 2002 guideline update for the management of patients with chronic stable angina—summary article: a report of the American College of Cardiology/American Heart Association Task Force on practice guidelines. *Journal of the American College of Cardiology, 41,* 159-168.

Grove, J. E., Bruscia, E. & Krause, D. S. (2004). Plasticity of bone marrow–derived stem cells. *Stem Cells, 22,* 487–500. doi: 10.1634/stemcells.22-4-48

Gulati, M., Cooper-DeHoff, R. M., McClure, C., Johnson, B. D., Shaw, L. J., Handberg, E. M., Zineh, I., ... & Bairey Merz, C.N. (2009). Adverse cardiovascular outcomes in women with nonobstructive coronary artery disease: A report from the women's ischemia syndrome evaluation study and the St James women take heart project. *Archives of Internal Medicine, 169*(9): 843-850.

Hallas, C. N., Wray, J., Andreou, P. & Banner, N.R. (2010). Depression and perceptions about heart failure predict quality of life in patients with advanced heart failure. *Heart & Lung: The Journal of Acute and Critical Care,* In Press, Corrected Proof. [Online] Available from: http://www.sciencedirect.com/science/article/B6WG7-4YT6NC4-7/2/2176f5f859b210a7507e9ed3a00e34b8

Haytowitz, D. B. & Bhagwat, S. (2010). USDA database for the oxygen radical absorbance capacity (ORAC) of selected foods, Release 2. Nutrient Data Laboratory. Retrieved from http://www.ars.usda.gov/SP2UserFiles/Place/12354500/Data/ORAC/ORAC_R2.pdf

Heiss, G., Wallace, R., Garnet, L., Anderson, G. L.,Aragaki, A., Beresford, S. A. A., Brzyski, R., ... & Stefanick, M. L., for the WHI Investigators (2008). Health risks and benefits 3 years after stopping randomized treatment with estrogen and progestin. *Journal of the American Medical Association, 299*(9), 1036-1045. doi: 10.1001/jama.299.9.1036

Heron, M., Hoyert, D. L, Murphy, S. L., Xu, J., Kochanek, K. D., & Tejada-Vera, B. (2009). National vital statistics reports. Retrieved from http://www.cdc.gov/nchs/data/nvsr/nvsr57/nvsr57_14.pdf

JAMA Patient Page Quality of Life (2002) JAMA patient quality of life. *Journal of the American Medical Association, 288*(23), 3070. [Online]. doi:10.1001/jama.288.23.3070 (Accessed: 9 February 2011).

Jiang, W. & Xiong, G. L. (2010). *Epidemiology of the comorbidity between depression and heart disease.* Chichester, UK: John Wiley & Sons, Ltd.

Johnstone, M. (1976). The effect of Lorazepam on the vasoconstriction of fear. *Anaesthesia, 31,* 868-872. doi: 10.1111/j.1365-2044.1976.tb11897.x

Kettawan, A., Kunthida, C., Takahashi, T., Kishi, T., Chikazawa, J., Sakata, Y., ... & Okamoto, T. (2007) The quality control assessment of commercially available coenzyme Q_{10}-containing dietary and health supplements in Japan, *Journal of Clinical Biochemistry Nutrition, 41*(2): 124–131. doi: 10.3164/jcbn.2007017

Kochar, P. G. (2004). What are stem cells? Retrieved from http://www.csa.com/discoveryguides/stemcell/overview.php

Krantz, D. S., Whittaker, K.S., Francis, J.L., Rutledge, T., Johnson, B. D., Barrow, G., ... & Bairey Merz, C.N. (2009) Epidemiology: Psychotropic medication use and risk of adverse cardiovascular events in women with suspected coronary artery disease: Outcomes from the Women's Ischemia Syndrome Evaluation (WISE) heart study, *95*, 1901-1906. doi:10.1136/hrt.2009.176040

Labos, C., Dasgupta, K., Nedjar, H., Turecki, G., & Rahme, E. (2011). Risk of bleeding associated with combined use of selective serotonin reuptake inhibitors and antiplatelet therapy following acute myocardial infarction. *Canadian Medical Association Journal.* cmaj.100912; published ahead of print September 26, 2011, doi:10.1503/cmaj.100912

Laino, C., (2005). Women with "normal" coronary arteries fare worse than men. *ESC 2005 Congress,* Abstracts 1642, 1430, 3468. Retrieved from http://www.medscape.com/viewarticle/512386

Langsjoen, P. H. (2002). The clinical use of HMG CoA-reductase inhibitors (statins) and the associated depletion of the essential co-factor coenzyme Q10: A review of pertinent human and animal data. FDA Docket, Exhibit A. http://www.fda.gov/ohrms/dockets/dailys/02/May02/052902/02p-0244-cp00001-02-Exhibit_A-vol1.pdf

Lloyd-Jones, D., Adams, R. J., Brown, T. M, Carnethon, M., Dai, S., De Simone, G., Ferguson, ... & Wylie-Rosett, J. and on behalf of the American Heart Association Statistics Committee and Stroke Statistics Subcommittee. (2010). Heart disease and stroke statistics—2010 update: A report from the American Heart Association. *Circulation, 121*(7), e46-e215. doi: 10.1161/CIRCULATIONAHA.109.192667

Lloyd-Jones, D., Adams, R., Carnethon, M., De Simone, Giovanni, Ferguson, T. B., Flegal, K., ... & Hong, Y., and for the American Heart Association Statistics Committee and Stroke Statistics Subcommittee. (2009). CHD and stroke statistics—2009 update—A report from the American Heart Association Statistics Committee and Stroke Statistics Subcommittee. doi: 10.1161/CIRCULATIONAHA.108.191261

Lunde, K., Solheim, S., Aakhus, S, Arnesen, H., Abdelnoor, M., & Forfang, K. (2005). Autologous stem cell transplantation in acute myocardial infarction: The ASTAMI randomized controlled trial, Intracoronary transplantation of autologous mononuclear bone marrow cells, study design and safety aspects. *Scandinavian Cardiovascular Journal, 39,* 150-158. doi: 10.1080/14017430510009131

McSweeney, J, C., Cody, M., O'Sullivan, P., Elberson, K., K. Moser, D.K., & Garvin, B.J. (2003) Women's early warning symptoms of acute myocardial infarction. *Circulation. 2003;108:2619-2623, published online before print November 3 2003,* doi:10.1161/01. CIR.0000097116.29625.7C

Mieres, J. H., Shaw, L. J., Arai, A., Budoff, M. J., Flamm, S. D., Hundley, W. G., Marwick, T. H., ... & Wenger, N. K.. (2005). Role of noninvasive testing in the clinical evaluation of women with suspected coronary artery disease: Consensus statement from the Cardiac Imaging Committee, Council on Clinical Cardiology, and the Cardiovascular Imaging and Intervention Committee, Council on Cardiovascular Radiology and Intervention, American Heart Association. *Circulation, 111,* 682-696. doi: 10.1161/01.CIR.0000155233.67287.60

Monteleone, P. (2010). The Association between depression and heart disease: The role of biological mechanisms in depression and heart disease. Chichester, UK: John Wiley & Sons, Ltd.

Morrison, M., & Samwick, A. A. (1940). Intramedullary (sternal) transfusion of human bone marrow. *Journal of the American Medical Association, 115,* 1708-1711. doi: 10.1001/ jama.1940.02810460040010

Mosca, L., Linfante, L. H., Benjamin, E. J.,Berra, K., Hayes, S. N., Walsh, B. W., Fabunmi, R. P., ... & Simpson, S. L. (2005). National study of physician awareness and adherence to cardiovascular disease prevention guidelines. *Circulation, 111,* 499-510. doi: 10.1161/01.CIR.0000154568.43333.82

Mosca, L., Banka, C. L., Benjamin, E. J., Berra, K., Bushnell, C., Dolor, R.J., Ganiats, T. G., ... & Wenger, N. K., and for the Expert Panel/Writing Group. (2007). Evidence-based guidelines for cardiovascular disease prevention in women: 2007 update. Circulation 115, 1481-501. doi: 10.1161/CIRCULA-TIONAHA.107.181546

National Institute of Health. (2009). Stem cell basics: Introduction. Retrieved from http://stemcells.nih.gov/info/basics/basics1

National Institute of Health. (2009). Stem Cell Basics: What are the similarities and differences between embryonic and adult stem cells? Retrieved from http://stemcells.nih.gov/info/basics/basics5

National Institute of Mental Health. (2002). *Anxiety Disorders* (NIH Publication No. 02-3879). Bethesda, MD: National Institute of Health.

Nielsen, F. H., Milne, D. B., Klevay, L. M., Gallagher, S., & Johnson, L. (2007). Dietary magnesium deficiency induces heart rhythm changes, impairs glucose tolerance, and decreases serum cholesterol in post-menopausal women. *Journal of American College of Nutrition, 26*(2), 121-132.

Ornish, D. (2010). Our genes are not our fate. In *This will change everything* (Ed. Brockman, J.). NY: HarperCollins.

Ornish D. (1992). Dr. Dean Ornish's program for reversing heart disease. NY: Ballantine Books.

Osgood, E. E., Riddle, M. C., & Mathews, T. J. (1939). Aplastic anemia treated with daily transfusions and intravenous marrow; case report. *American Journal of Medicine, 13*, 357–367. DOI:10.1059/0003-4819-13-2-357

Paajanen T. A., Oksala N. K., Kuukasjärvi P. & Karhunen, P. J. (2010). Short stature is associated with coronary heart disease: a systematic review of the literature and a meta-analysis. *European Heart Journal, 31*, 1802–1809. doi:10.1093/eurheartj/ehq155

Pan, A., Lucas, M., Sun, Q., van Dam, R., M., Franco, O. H., Willett, W. C., Manson, J. E., ... & Hu, F. B. (2011). Increased mortality risk in women with depression and diabetes mellitus. *Archives of General Psychiatry 69*, 42-50. Retrieved from http://archpsyc. ama-assn.org/cgi/content/abstract/68/1/42

Patel, A. N., Geffner, L., Vina, R. F., Saslavsky, J., Urschel, H. C., Jr, Kormos, R., & Benetti, F. (2005). Surgical treatment for congestive heart failure with autologous adult stem cell transplantation: A prospective randomized study. *Journal of Thoracic Cardiovascular Surgery, 130*, 1631-1638. doi: 10.1016/j. jtcvs.2005.07.056

Pedersen, S. S., Herrmann-Lingen, C., de Jonge, P., & Scherer, M. (2010). Type D personality is a predictor of poor emotional quality of life in primary care heart failure patients independent of depressive symptoms and New York Heart Association functional class. *Journal of Behavioral Medicine, (33)*1. [Online]. Available from: http://www.metapress.com. ezproxy.liv.ac.uk/content/a0067x173332xw72/

Perin, E. C., Dohmann, H. F. R., Borojevic, R., Silva, S. A., Sousa, A. L. S., Mesquita, C. T., ... & Prior, R. L., Joseph, J. A., Cao, G., & Shukitt-Hale, B. (1999). Can foods forestall aging? *Agricult Res. 47*(2):14-17.

Pritikin, N., Leonard, J. & Hofer, J. L. (1974). *Live longer now: The first 100 years of your life.* New York: Grosset & Dunlap.

Pritikin, N. & McGrady, P. M. (1979). *The Pritikin program for diet and exercise.* New York: Grosset & Dunlap.

Quality Metrics. (2011). SF 36v2 Health Survey. Retrieved from http://www.qualitymetric.com/Portals/0/Uploads/Documents/Public/SF-36v2%20Health%20Survey%20Measurement%20Model.pdf

Regents of the University of Minnesota. (2010). Minnesota living with heart failure questionnaire. Retrieved from http://www.license.umn.edu/Products/Minnesota-Living-With-Heart-Failure-Questionnaire__Z94019.aspx

Rekers, P. E., Coulter, M. P., & Warren, S. L. (1950). Effect of transplantation of bone marrow into irradiated animals. *Archives of Surgery, 60*(4), 635-667. Retrieved from http://archsurg.ama-assn.org/cgi/reprint/60/4/635

Rich, M. W., Beckham, V., Wittenberg, C., Leven, C. L., Freedland, K. E., & Carney, R. M. (1995). A multidisciplinary intervention to prevent the readmission of elderly patients with congestive heart failure. *New England Journal of Medicine, 333*(18):1190-5. [Online]. Available from: http://content.nejm.org/cgi/content/full/333/18/1190

Rich-Edwards, J. W., Manson, J. E., Stampfer, M. J., Colditz, G. A., Willett, W. C, Rosner. B., Speizer, F. E., & Hennekens, C. H. (1995). Height and the risk of cardiovascular disease in women. *American Journal of Epidemiology, (142)*9, 909-917, Retrieved from http://aje.oxfordjournals.org/content/142/9/909.abstract?ijkey=a445d3f8c2d3b50e8ff1044226c23b71f1d58db3&keytype2=tf_ipsecsha

Ridker, P. M., Cook, N. R., Lee, I. M., Gordon, D., Gaziano, J. M., Manson, J. E., ... & Buring, J. E. (2005). A randomized trial of low-dose aspirin in the primary prevention of cardiovascular disease in women. *New England Journal of Medicine, 352*, 1293-1304. Retrieved from http://www.nejm.org/doi/full/10.1056/NEJMoa050613

Ring, L., Hofer, S., Heuston, F., Harris, D., & O'Boyle, C. (2005). Response shift masks the treatment impact on patient reported outcomes (PROs): The example of individual. Retrieved from http://www.hqlo.com/content/pdf/1477-7525-3-55.pdf

Roger, V. L., Go, A. S., Lloyd-Jones, D. M., Adams, R. J., Berry, J. D., Brown, T. M., Carnethon, M. R., & Wylie-Rosett, J. (2011). Heart disease and stroke statistics—2011 update: A report from the American Heart Association. *Circulation 123*, 18–209. doi: 10.1161/CIR.0b013e3182009701

Roncalli, J., Mouquet, F., Piot, C., Trochu, J. N., Corvoisier, P. L., Neuder, Y., ... & Lemarchand, P. (2010). Intracoronary autologous mononucleated bone marrow cell infusion for acute myocardial infarction: Results of the randomized multicenter BONAMI trial. *European Heart Journal.* doi:10.1093/eurheartj/ehq455

Rosch, P. J. (1989) "Stress addiction": Causes, consequences, and cures. In Flach, F. (Ed). *Stress and its management* (pp.189-202). New York: Norton.

Rosenfeld, L. (1992). *Yale heart book: Women and heart disease* (Chapter 9.) 237-246. Retrieved from http://www.med.yale.edu/library/heartbk/19.pdf

Sackett, D. L., Rosenberg, W. M. C., Gray, J. A. M., Haynes, R. B., & Richardson, W., S. (1996). Evidence based medicine: What it's and what it'sn't. *British Medical Journal 312*, 71-72. Retrieved from http://www.bmj.com/content/312/7023/71.full

Schipper, H. (1983). Why measure quality of life? *Canadian Medical Association Journal,* 128 Retrieved from http://www.ncbi.nlm.nih.gov/pmc/articles/PMC1875788/pdf/canmedaj01393-0062.pdf

Schächinger, V., Erbs, S., Elsässer, A., Haberbosch, W., Hambrecht, R., Hölschermann, H., ... & Zeiher, A. M. (2006). Intracoronary bone marrow—Derived progenitor cells in acute myocardial infarction. *New England Journal of Medicine, 355*, 1210-1221. doi: 10.1056/NEJMoa060186

Sears, S. F., Serber, E. R., Lewis, T. S., Walker, R. L., Conners, N., Lee, J. T., Curtis, A. B., Conti, J. B. (2004), Do positive health expectations and optimism relate to quality-of-life outcomes for the patient with an implantable cardioverter defibrillator? *Journal of Cardiopulmonary Rehabilitation,* 24(5):324-31. [Online]. Available from: http://journals.lww.com/jcrjournal/Abstract/2004/09000/Do_Positive_Health_Expectations_and_Optimism.8.aspx

Shaw, L. J., Bairey Merz, C. N., Pepine, C. J., Reis, S.E, Bittner, V., Kelsey, S.F., Olson, M., ... & Sopko, G. for the WISE Investigators. (2006). Insights from the NHLBI-sponsored women's ischemia syndrome evaluation study: Part I: Gender differences in traditional and novel risk factors, symptom evaluation, and gender-optimized diagnostic strategies. *Journal of the American College of Cardiology, 47,* S4-S20.

Silva, G. V., Perin, E. C., Dohmann, H. F., Borojevic, R., Silva, S. A., Sousa, A. L., Assad, J. A., ... & Willerson, J. T. (2004). Catheter-based transendocardial delivery of autologous bone-marrow-derived mononuclear cells in patients listed for heart transplantation. *Texas Heart Institute Journal,.* 31(3), 214–219. Retrieved from http://www.ncbi.nlm.nih.gov/pmc/articles/PMC521759/

Sinha, I. P., Smyth, R. L., & Williamson, P. R. (2011). Using the delphi technique to determine which outcomes to measure in clinical trials: Recommendations for the future based on a systematic review of existing studies. *PLoS Medicine, 8,* 1. doi:10.1371/journal.pmed.1000393

Slopen, N., Glynn, R. J., Buring, J., and Albert, M. A. (2010). Promoting cardiovascular health: Decreasing risk and increasing physical activity abstract, Job strain, job insecurity, and incident cardiovascular disease in the women's health study. (Presentation). Retrieved from http://www.abstractsonline.com/Plan/ViewAbstract.aspx?sKey=5f95496c-7c94-4b4d-9481-c544808d59ed&cKey=298a847c-bbad-467c-8308-bd6990c73502&mKey=%7bFAD5CF04-7CC9-470A-8A02-B69A7E5EA4F3%7d

Strauer, B. E., Brehm, M., Zeus, T., Köstering, M., Hernandez, A., Sorg, R. V., ... & Wernet, P. (2002). Repair of infarcted myocardium by autologous intracoronary mononuclear bone marrow cell transplantation in humans. *Circulation, 106,* 1913-1918. Retrieved from http://circ.ahajournals.org/cgi/reprint/106/15/1913

Sumi, H., Hamada, H., Tsushima, H., Mihara, H., Muraki, H. (1987). *Experientia, 15*(43), 1110-1111.

Suzuki, Y., Kondo, K., Ichise, H., Tsukamoto, Y., Urano, T., & Umemura, K. (2003). Dietary supplementation with fermented soybeans suppresses intimal thickening. *Nutrition, 19*(3), 261-264.

Testa, M. A., & Simonson, D. C. (1996). Assessment of quality-of-life outcomes. *New England Journal of Medicine, 334,* 835-840. Retrieved from http://www.nejm.org/doi/pdf/10.1056/NEJM199603283341306

The ENRICHD Investigators. (2001) Enhancing Recovery in Coronary Heart Disease (ENRICHD) Study Intervention: Rationale and Design *Psychosomatic Medicine, 63,* 747-755. http://www.psychosomaticmedicine.org/content/63/5/747.full#

The Lancet. (2011). Cardiovascular disease in women—Often silent and fatal. *The Lancet, 378*(9787), 200. doi: 10.1016/S0140-6736(11)61108-2

Thomas, D. E., (1990). Bone marrow transplantation—Past, present and future, (Nobel Lecture). Retrieved from http://nobelprize.org/nobel_prizes/medicine/laureates/1990/thomas-lecture.pdf

Tobin, J. N., Wassertheil-Smoller, S., Wexler, J. P., Steingart, R. M., Budner, N., Lense, L., & Wachspress, J. (1987). Sex bias in considering coronary bypass surgery. *Annals of Internal Medicine, 107*, 19-25.

Tran, M. T., Mitchell, T. M., Kennedy, D. T., & Giles, J. T. (2001) Role of coenzyme Q10 in chronic heart failure, angina, and hypertension. *Pharmacotherapy, 21*, 797–806.

U. S. Census Bureau Division. (2010). Retrieved from http://www.census.gov/population/www/socdemo/age/general-age.html#bb

U. S. Census Bureau. (2010). About Us. Retrieved from http://www.census.gov/aboutus/

U. S. Department of Health & Human Service. (2010). The Health Insurance Portability and Accountability Act of 1996 (HIPAA) Privacy and Security Rules. Retrieved from http://www.hhs.gov/ocr/privacy/hipaa/understanding/index.html

U. S. National Library of Medicine. (1999). MEDLINE. Retrieved from http://www.nlm.nih.gov/databases/databases_medline.html

U. S. Patent 4 933 165. June 12, 1990. Coenzyme Q.sub.10 with HMG-CoA reductase inhibitors. A pharmaceutical composition and method of counteracting HMG-CoA reductase inhibitor-associated myopathy is disclosed. The method comprises the adjunct administration of an effective amount of an HMG-CoA reductase inhibitor and an effective amount of coenzyme Q.sub.10. Inventors: Brown MS (Dallas, TX). Assignee: Merck & Co Inc (Rahway, NJ).

U. S. Patent 4 929 437. May 29, 1990. Coenzyme Q sub 10 with HMG-CoA reductase inhibitors. A pharmaceutical composition and method of counteracting HMG-CoA reductase inhibitor-associated elevated transaminase levels is disclosed. The method comprises the adjunct administration of an effective amount of an HMG-CoA reductase inhibitor and an effective amount of coenzyme Q sub10. Inventors: Tobert, J. A. (Maplewood, NJ). Assignee: Merck & Co., Inc. (Rahway, NJ).

University of Liverpool. (2010). COMET initiative. Retrieved from http://www.liv.ac.uk/nwhtmr/research/theme_2/core_outcomes.htm

University of Minnesota. (2010). Minnesota living with heart failure questionnaire. Retrieved from http://www.license.umn.edu/Products/Minnesota-Living-With-Heart-Failure-Questionnaire__Z94019.aspx

University of Oxford. (2008). Patient reported outcome measurement group, instrument types. Retrieved from http://phi.uhce.ox.ac.uk/inst_types.php (Accessed: 28 January 2011).

Wain, L. V., Verwoert, G. C., O'Reilly, P. F., Shi, G., Johnson, T., Johnson, A. D., Bochud, M., ... & van Duijn, C. M. (2011). Genome-wide association study identifies six new loci influencing pulse pressure and mean arterial pressure. *Nature Genetics, 43*:1005-1011.

Watkins, L. L., Schneiderman, N., Blumenthal, J. A., Sheps, D. S., Catellier, D., Taylor,C.B., & Freedland, K. E. (2003). Cognitive and somatic symptoms of depression are associated with medical comorbidity in patients after acute myocardial infarction. *American Heart Journal, 146*, 48-54. [Online] doi: 10.1016/S0002-8703(03)00083-8

Wei, H. M., Wong P, Hsu L F, & Shim W. (2009). Human bone marrow-derived adult stem cells for post-myocardial infarction cardiac repair: Current status and future directions. *Singapore Medical Journal Review, 50*, 10, 935. Retrieved from http://smj.sma.org.sg/5010/5010ra1.pdf

Whang, W., Kubzansky, L. D., Kawachi, I., Rexrode, K. M., Kroenke, C. H., Glynn, R. J., ... & Albert, C. M. (2009). Depression and risk of sudden cardiac death and coronary heart disease in women: Results from the nurses' health study. *Journal of the American College of Cardiology, 53*, 950-958.

Willerson, J. T. , Perin , E. C., Ellis, S. G., Pepine, C. J., Henry, T. D., Zhao, D. X. M., ... & Simari, R. D. (2010). Intramyocardial injection of autologous bone marrow mononuclear cells for patients with chronic ischemic heart disease and left ventricular dysfunction (First Mononuclear Cells injected in the US [FOCUS]): Rationale and design. *American Heart Journal, 160*(2), 215-223. Retrieved from http://www.sciencedirect.com/science/article/B6W9H-50PKK8G-5/2/5204f41fa6f022 4de75fea9a46eb65b7

Witschi, A., Reddy, S., Stofer, B. and Lauterburg, B. (1992). The systemic availability of oral glutathione. *European Journal of Clinical Pharmacology, 43*(6), 667-669 [Online] doi: 10.1007/ BF02284971

Wollert, K. C., Meyer, G. P., Lotz, J., Lichtenberg, S. R., Lippolt, P., Breidenbach, C., ... & Drexler, H. (2004). Intracoronary autologous bone-marrow cell transfer after myocardial infarction: The BOOST randomized controlled clinical trial, *The Lancet, 364*(9429), 141-148. doi: 10.1016/S0140-6736(04)16626-9

World Health Organization. (2011). About WHO. Retrieved from http://www.who.int/en/

World Health Organization. (1997). Measuring quality of life. Retrieved from http://www.who.int/mental_health/ media/68.pdf

Wulff, H. (1999). The two cultures of medicine: Objective facts versus subjectivity and values. *Journal of Royal Society of Medi-*

cine, 92. Retrieved from http://www.ncbi.nlm.nih.gov/pmc/articles/PMC1297426/pdf/jrsocmed00003-0007.pdf

Xu, J., Kochanek, K., Murphy, S. L., & Tejada-Vera, B. (2010). Deaths: Final data for 2007. *National Vital Statistics Reports, 58*, 19. Retrieved from http://www.cdc.gov/nchs/data/nvsr/nvsr58/nvsr58_19.pdf.

Yousef, M., Schannwell, C. M., Köstering, M., Zeus, T., Brehm, M., & Strauer, B. E. (2009). The BALANCE study: Clinical benefit and long-term outcome after intracoronary autologous bone marrow cell transplantation in patients with acute myocardial infarction. *Journal of the American College of Cardiology, 53*, 2262-2269. doi: 10.1016/j.jacc.2009.02.051

For more information on Cardiovascular Stem Cells and Clinical Trials, see:

NIH Clinical Trial for Congestive Heart Failure http://clinicaltrial.gov/ct2/results?term=stem+cell+%2B+congestive+heart+failure

NIH Clinical Trial for Heart Attack (MI)

http://clinicaltrial.gov/ct2/results?term=stem+cell+%2B+heart+attack

NIH Clinical Trial for Cardiomyopathy

http://clinicaltrial.gov/ct2/results?term=stem+cell+%2B+cardiomyopathy

NIH Clinical Trial for Coronary Artery Disease (CAD)

http://clinicaltrial.gov/ct2/results?term=stem+cell+%2B+coronary+artery+disease

NIH Clinical Trial for Peripheral Artery Disease (PAD)

http://clinicaltrial.gov/ct2/results?term=stem+cell+%2B+peripheral+artery+disease

PMA BIBLIOGRAPHY:

Compiled by Judith Williamson

1. Definiteness of Purpose:
   Your Greatest Power
   > J. Martin Kohe

   The Artist's Way
   Vein of Gold
   > Julia Cameron

2. The Master Mind:
   Seabiscuit: An American Legend
   > Laura Hillenbrand

3. Applied Faith
   Believe and Achieve
   > W. Clement Stone

   The Magic of Believing
   TNT: The Power Within You
   > Claude M. Bristol

4. Going the Extra Mile
   Try Giving Yourself Away
   > David Dunn

The Greatest Salesman in the World
Og Mandino

5. Pleasing Personality
How to Win Friends and Influence People
Dale Carnegie

6. Personal Initiative:
The Success System That Never Fails
W. Clement Stone

The Alchemist
Paulo Coelho

7. Positive Mental Attitude:
The Power of Positive Thinking
Norman Vincent Peale

Man's Search for Meaning
Victor Frankl

Love, Medicine & Miracles
Peace, Love and Healing
Bernie S. Siegel, M.D.

8. Enthusiasm:
Life is Tremendous
Charlie T. Jones

9. Self-Discipline:
A Message to Garcia
Elbert Hubbard

10. Accurate Thinking:
Key to Yourself

Venice Bloodworth

11. Controlled Attention:
As A Man Thinketh
James Allen

12. Teamwork:
The Wonderful Wizard of Oz
L. Frank Baum

13. Learning from Adversity and Defeat:
Acres of Diamonds
R. H. Conwell

The Anatomy of Hope: How People Prevail in the Face of Illness
Dr. Jerome Groopman

14. Creative Vision:
Your Word is Your Wand
Florence Scovel Shinn

The Richest Man of Babylon
George S. Clason

15. Maintenance of Sound Health:
Wake Up! You're Alive
Arnold Fox, M.D. & Barry Fox, Ph.D

Ancient Secret of the Fountain of Youth, Book 1
Ancient Secret of the Fountain of Youth, Book 2
Peter Kelder

16. Budgeting Time and Money:
Seven Habits of Highly Effective People

Stephen R. Covey

17. Cosmic Habitforce:
The Power of Your Subconscious Mind
Dr. Joseph Murphy

About the Book

D r. Dori Naerbo has a personal reason for concern about the female heart. After three consecutive heart attacks, she was numb, depressed and paralyzed with fear as a fourth heart attack loomed like a thundercloud over head. Her doctors were puzzled since they could not determine the cause, nor could they give a prognosis. Naerbo knew that she had to take charge to prevent the next attack.

Out of this healing journey she wrote an inspirational and motivating story, **"A Women's Heart Attack: What Your Doctor May Not Tell You"**, sharing her step-by-step process, supported by science and research focused on three important areas (body, mind and spirit). As an autologous stem cell consultant and advocate, she has spoken to thousands of cardiac patients and gleaned important information, together, with her experiences she provides you with insights about healing your heart. This book is for all women or anyone concerned about a special woman—a partner, wife, sister, mother, aunt, grandmother, cousin, friend, or colleague.

"At my last cardiovascular visit, my doctor said, You've completely healed yourself. I can see no evidence that you've had a heart attack," Naerbo remembers.

Here are just a few things you will learn:

♥ Gender differences and why the medical establishment treats women differently than men.

💜 Power descriptors without them you can be referred to a psychiatrist or gastroenterologist, when you really need a cardiologist!

💜 Risk factors specific to women.

💜 Early warnings signs, which can present one month before an attack.

💜 How to use your body/mind/spirit as one to achieve healing and recovery.

💜 Astonishing connection between hormones that renders women vulnerable to heart attacks.

Most important, you will learn how Dr. Dori completely healed herself and transformed her life. She explains these factors in detail to empower you toward your own good health and much more. There is life after a heart attack regardless of gender. Women, you do have the power to heal yourself. Read *A Woman's Heart Attack: What Your Doctor May Not Tell You* to find out how.

BIO

Dori Naerbo, Ph.D., Org.Psy. MSc., Clinical Research from the University of Liverpool, is a consultant for biotech companies, and clinical researcher with a special interest in autologous stem cells and its cardiovascular applications. She is a native Californian who now lives in Norway with her husband of 32 years. She travels the world spreading her message of hope and healing to all women. (www.dorinaerbo.com)

18162798R00159

Made in the USA
Charleston, SC
20 March 2013